Other monographs in the series, Major Problems in Clinical Surgery

Child, et al.; *The Liver and Portal Hypertension*

Welch: *Polypoid Lesions of the Gastrointestinal Tract*

Madding and Kennedy: *Trauma to the Liver* (Second Edition)

Barker: *Peripheral Arterial Disease*

Spratt and Donegan: *Cancer of the Breast*

Haller: *Deep Thrombophlebitis*

Colcock and Braasch: *Surgery of the Small Intestine in the Adult*

Jackman and Beahrs: *Tumors of the Large Bowel*

Ellis and Olsen: *Achalasia of the Esophagus*

Botsford and Wilson: *The Acute Abdomen*

Colcock: *Diverticular Disease of the Colon*

Spratt, Butcher and Bricker: *Exenterative Surgery of the Pelvis*

Child: *Portal Hypertension*

Sedgwick: *Surgery of the Thyroid Gland*

SHOCK

by

G. Tom Shires, M.D.

Professor and Chairman, Department of
Surgery, The University of Texas Southwestern Medical School at Dallas

Charles J. Carrico, M.D.

Associate Professor, Department of Surgery, The
University of Texas Southwestern Medical School
at Dallas

Peter C. Canizaro, M.D.

Associate Professor, Department of Surgery,
The University of Texas Southwestern Medical
School at Dallas

Volume XIII in the Series

**MAJOR PROBLEMS IN
CLINICAL SURGERY**

J. ENGLEBERT DUNPHY, M.D.
Consulting Editor

W. B. Saunders Company   Philadelphia, London, Toronto, 1973

3 / 2

W. B. Saunders Company: West Washington Square
Philadelphia, Pa. 19105

12 Dyott Street
London, WC1A   1DB

833 Oxford Street
Toronto 18, Ontario

Shock   ISBN 0-7216-8250-2

Print No.:   9   8   7   6   5   4   3   2   1

Foreword

Dr. Tom Shires and his group were asked to prepare this monograph on shock because not only have they had a long and scholarly interest in research in this field, but this interest has been combined with an intense and practical clinical experience. The reader will find this dual interest manifest throughout the book. Experimental studies on fluid replacement, electrolyte changes, renal function, oxygen transport and cellular membrane potential provide the basis for a critical and sophisticated analysis of each aspect of the problem as seen clinically. Upon this basis the authors have built a logical approach to therapy.

It is gratifying to see that the sound classification of shock presented by Alfred Blalock in 1940 is used by the authors. Although cardiogenic, neurogenic and septic shock are dealt with in a separate chapter, each aspect of these varied types of shock is integrated into the practical care of the patient. The gravity and extent of modern injury, the frequency of superimposed sepsis and the cardiac problems of the elderly present combined problems in a vast majority of cases. The authors deal with this in a very practical way in their section on therapy.

This monograph combines all the advantages of a sophisticated scientific work of reference with practical daily applications. It should prove to be a "vade mecum" for all who work in emergency wards or deal with the complex problems of shock.

J. ENGLEBERT DUNPHY, M.D.

Preface

This work on shock is an attempt to briefly compile an overview of the major problems associated with the consequences of severe bodily injury. These problems have been categorized into three major areas for discussion: (1) clinical manifestations, (2) pathophysiologic responses and (3) therapy. The various types of shock are dealt with in each of these categories. It is hoped that this will provide a useful and logical approach to the often encountered symptom complex called "shock."

An attempt has also been made to collate the newer and more sophisticated research knowledge in several specific areas. It should be clear that the effects of shock on cellular function are being more carefully examined.

The authors have been working with the clinical and laboratory aspects of this symptom complex for several years. Much of the work presented could not have been done without the valuable assistance of a number of fellows, residents, research associates and technicians over the years. In addition, the Trauma Research Unit, funded by the National Institute of General Medical Sciences of the National Institutes of Health, has been of inestimable value in the collection of data on seriously injured patients. The fellows, house staff, research nurses and technicians in this unit are responsible for studies on patients which have never been gathered previously.

The more recent contributors to various sections of these continuing studies include:

Chapters 1, 2 and 6: Dr. G. Tom Shires, Dr. Donald Trunkey, Dr. Ronald Holliday, Dr. Joseph P. Cunningham, Dr. Steven Reeder, Dr. Richard Baker and Dr. Hana Illner.

Chapter 3: Dr. Charles Baxter and Dr. Richard Baker.

Chapter 4: Dr. Charles Carrico, Dr. Joel Horovitz and Dr. Lewis Flint.

Chapter 5: Dr. Peter Canizaro, Dr. James Nelson and John Hennessy.

Chapter 7: Dr. Peter Canizaro, Dr. Charles Carrico and Dr. Winfred Sugg.

Research Associates who aided us include Jan Maher, Yvonne Wagner, Ginger Miller, Becky Backof, Sheryl Kappus, Mary Ann Edgar, Bill Purcell, Janet Marvin, R.N., John Hicks and Melvin Vaught.

The authors would also like to express their appreciation to Betty McSpedden, Jean Gross and Ila Fite for secretarial and editorial assistance.

G. TOM SHIRES
CHARLES J. CARRICO
PETER C. CANIZARO

Contents

Section I
CLINICAL MANIFESTATIONS OF SHOCK

Chapter 1

CLASSIFICATION AND CLINICAL AND PHYSIOLOGIC
MANIFESTATIONS OF SHOCK 3

Definition and Working Classification 3
Physiologic Changes 7
    Blood Pressure 7
    Pulse Rate... 7
    Vasoconstriction 8
    Hemodilution... 8
Biochemical Changes.. 9
    Pituitary-Adrenal 9
    Low-Flow State 10
    Organ Failure 11
References... 11

Section II
PATHOPHYSIOLOGIC RESPONSES TO SHOCK

Chapter 2

RESPONSE OF THE EXTRACELLULAR FLUID 15

Experimental Studies.. 15
    Early Results 15
    Recent Cellular Studies.. 18
        Small Animal Studies... 19
        Subhuman Primate Studies.................................. 25
        Interpretation of Experimental Studies 33
        Other Evidence of Cellular Response.................... 35
        Summary.. 40
References... 40

Chapter 3

RENAL RESPONSES 42

Subclinical Renal Damage Following Injury and Shock 42
    Patient Studies 43
    Discussion 46
High-Output Renal Failure 50
    Patient Studies 50
    Animal Studies 56
    Discussion 58
References 59

Chapter 4

PULMONARY RESPONSES 61

Clinical Presentation 62
    Phase I: Injury, Resuscitation and Alkalosis 62
    Phase II: Circulatory Stabilization and Beginning
        Respiratory Difficulty 62
    Phase III: Progressive Pulmonary Insufficiency 63
    Phase IV: Terminal Hypoxia and Hypercarbia
        with Asystole 63
Etiology 64
    Hemorrhagic Shock (Ischemic Pulmonary Injury) 65
    Pulmonary Infection 69
    Sepsis 70
    Aspiration 70
    Fat Embolization 71
    Microembolization 71
    Fluid Overload 72
    Oxygen Toxicity 75
    Microatelectasis 76
    Direct Pulmonary Injury 76
    Cerebral Injury 76
Mechanism 77
    Hypoxia 77
Treatment 80
    Patient Monitoring 82
        Evaluation of Oxygenation 82
        Assessment of Ventilation 84
        Evaluation of Pulmonary Mechanics 84
        Indications for Therapy 84
    Ventilatory Support 85
        General 85
        Control of P_{CO_2} 87

Constant Positive-Pressure Breathing (CPPB) 87
Complications.. 88
Fluid Management.. 89
Pulmonary Care 90
Drugs.. 90
Diuretics.. 91
Steroids.. 91
Heparin 91
Antibiotics 92
Summary.. 92
References.. 92

Chapter 5

ALTERATIONS IN OXYGEN TRANSPORT 97

Oxygen Transport 97
Oxygen-Hemoglobin Dissociation Curve............................ 99
Factors Influencing the Position of the Oxygen-
Hemoglobin Dissociation Curve 101
Blood Transfusions, Erythrocyte DPG and
Oxygen Delivery.. 104
Therapeutic Implications 109
References.. 114

Section III
THERAPY OF SHOCK

Chapter 6

HYPOVOLEMIC SHOCK 119

Volume.. 120
Extracellular Fluid Replacement............................ 120
Blood Transfusions.. 121
Hematocrit 124
Blood Substitutes 125
Positioning.. 126
Pulmonary Support.. 127
Antibiotics 128
Treatment of Pain 128
Steroids.. 129
Digitalis.. 129
Intra-arterial Infusions 129
Hypothermia.. 130
Renal Hypothermia.. 135
Vasopressors 135

Vasodilators 137
Hemodynamic Measurements 138
References 141

Chapter 7

CARDIOGENIC, NEUROGENIC, AND SEPTIC SHOCK 145

Cardiogenic Shock 145
    Hemodynamic Measurements 145
    Abnormalities in Contractility 147
        Digitalis 147
        Catecholamines 147
        Ganglionic Blockade 148
    Abnormalities in Rate 148
        Rapid Ventricular Rates 148
        Low Output 149
    Mechanical Assistance 149
Neurogenic Shock 149
Septic Shock 151
    Gram-Positive Sepsis and Shock 151
    Gram-Negative Sepsis and Shock 152
        Source 152
        Associated Conditions 152
        Bacteriology 153
        Clinical Manifestations 153
        Treatment 156
            Antibiotic Therapy 156
            Fluid Replacement 157
            Steroids 158
            Vasoactive Drugs 158
            Digitalis 159
            Pulmonary Therapy 160
References 160

INDEX 163

SECTION

I

Clinical
Manifestations
of Shock

Chapter One

CLASSIFICATION AND CLINICAL AND PHYSIOLOGIC MANIFES-TATIONS OF SHOCK

DEFINITION AND WORKING CLASSIFICATION

The scope of modern medicine is increasing steadily. As understanding of physiologic and biochemical derangements is broadened, so is the horizon of possibilities for the relief of illness. As more seriously ill patients are presented, shock is a symptom complex more frequently encountered by the physician.

Although shock has been recognized for over 100 years, a clear definition and dissection of this complex and devastating state has emerged only slowly. Many attempts have been made over the years to define adequately the entity known as shock. In 1872 the elder Gross defined shock as a "manifestation of the rude unhinging of the machinery of life."[8] Although the accuracy of this definition is unquestioned, it is obviously far from precise. In 1942 Wiggers, on the basis of an exhaustive examination of available evidence at that time, offered the definition: "Shock is a syndrome resulting from a depression of many functions, but in which reduction of the effective circulating blood volume is of basic importance, and in which impairment of the circulation steadily progresses until it eventuates in a state of irreversible circulatory failure."[18] A definition which Blalock

3

offered in 1940 was that "Shock is a peripheral circulatory failure, resulting from a discrepancy in the size of the vascular bed and the volume of the intravascular fluid."[2]

A more modern definition has been devised by Simeone.[15] He stated that shock may be defined as a "clinical condition characterized by signs and symptoms which arise when the cardiac output is insufficient to fill the arterial tree with blood under sufficient pressure to provide organs and tissues with adequate blood flow."

Shock of all forms appears to be invariably related to inadequate tissue perfusion. The low-flow state in vital organs seems to be the final common denominator in all forms of shock.

For purposes of a working clinical classification, the etiologic classification offered by Blalock in 1934 is still a useful and functional one.[3] Blalock suggested four categories:

1. Hematogenic (oligemia)
2. Neurogenic (caused primarily by nervous influences)
3. Vasogenic (initially decreased vascular resistance and increased vascular capacity)
4. Cardiogenic
   a. Failure of the heart as a pump
   b. Unclassified category (including diminished cardiac output from various causes)

It is now clear that shock invariably results from loss of function of one or more of four separate but interrelated functions. These are:

1. The pump (heart)
2. The fluid which is pumped (blood volume)
3. Arteriolar resistance vessels
4. The capacity of the venous bed (capacitance vessels)

In the context of Blalock's etiologic classification, these functions may be correlated:

1. Cardiogenic shock. This implies failure of the heart as a pump and may be brought about by:
   a. Primary myocardial dysfunction from
      (1) Myocardial infarction
      (2) Serious cardiac arrhythmias
      (3) Myocardial depression from a variety of causes
   b. Miscellaneous causes would include mechanical restriction of cardiac function or venous obstruction such as occurs in the mediastinum with:
      (1) Tension pneumothorax
      (2) Vena caval obstruction
      (3) Cardiac tamponade

2. Reduction in the fluid which may be pumped, the blood volume. This loss of volume may be in the form of loss of whole blood, plasma or extracellular fluid in the extravascular space, or a combination of these three.

3. Changes in resistance vessels may be brought about by specific disorders, which would include:
    a. Decrease in resistance
        (1) Spinal anesthesia
        (2) Neurogenic reflexes, as in acute pain
        (3) Possibly the end stages of hypovolemic shock
    b. Septic shock
        (1) Change in peripheral arterial resistance
        (2) Change in venous capacitance
        (3) Peripheral arteriovenous shunting

Therapy of shock will obviously revolve around the etiologic type or combination of types of shock present in a given patient who has undergone trauma.

The signs and symptoms of hypovolemic shock, when they are well established, are classic and usually easy to recognize. Most of the signs of clinical shock are characteristic of low peripheral blood flow and are contributed to by the effects of excess adrenal-sympathetic activity. The signs and symptoms of shock in man, according to the severity of the shock, were well described by Beecher et al., as summarized in Table 1-1.

On first inspection the patient in shock presents an anxious, tired expression, which early is that of restlessness and anxiety and later becomes a picture of apathy or exhaustion. Typically, the skin feels cool and is pale and mottled, and there is evidence of decreased capillary flow exhibited by easy blanching of the skin, particularly the nail beds.

Table 1-1   Grading of Shock

			SKIN				
DEGREE OF SHOCK	BLOOD PRESSURE (APPROX.)	PULSE QUALITY	TEM-PERATURE	COLOR	CIRCULATION (RESPONSE TO PRESSURE BLANCHING)	THIRST	MENTAL STATE
None	Normal	Normal	Normal	Normal	Normal	Normal	Clear and distressed
Slight	To 20% increase	Normal	Cool	Pale	Definite slowing	Normal	Clear and distressed
Moderate	Decreased 20–40%	Definite decrease in volume	Cool	Pale	Definite slowing	Definite	Clear and some apathy unless stimulated
Severe	Decreased 40% to non-recordable	Weak to imperceptible	Cold	Ashen to cyanotic (mottling)	Very sluggish	Severe	Apathetic to comatose, little distress except thirst

From H. K. Beecher, F. A. Simeone, C. H. Burnett, S. L. Shapiro, E. R. Sullivan and T. B. Mallory: The internal state of the severely wounded man on entry to the most forward hospital. Surgery, 22:672, 1947.

There are varying discrepancies in the classic picture of shock. In neurogenic shock, particularly that in response to spinal anesthesia, the pulse rate is normal or, more often, decreased; the pulse pressure is wide, and the pulse feels strong rather than weak. The rapid pulse characteristic of early hemorrhagic or wound shock may be absent, even if the patient has lost blood rapidly. This is also true if his position is supine or prone, in which case a rapid pulse may not appear until the patient is moved or elevated to a sitting position.[13] The varying clinical picture in septic shock is discussed in Chapter Seven.

In observing a large number of patients in hemorrhagic hypovolemic shock, one sees remarkably varied but typical responses of the sensorium to the shock episode. Most young, healthy patients who sustain wound or hemorrhagic shock, when seen early after the wounding, will appear to be restless and anxious and actually give the appearance of great fear. Shortly after being seen by a physician and started on treatment, this restlessness frequently gives way to great apathy, and the patient will appear sleepy. When aroused, he may complain of weakness or of a chilly sensation, although he does not actually have a chill. If blood loss is unchecked, the patient's apathy and sleepiness will rapidly progress into coma. In treating a large number of accident victims, it has been our experience that a patient who has bled into frank coma from which he cannot be aroused, resulting simply from blood loss alone (unassociated with other injuries such as brain damage), has usually sustained lethal blood loss. This sign usually indicates rapid massive hemorrhage for which the compensations to shock are inadequate to maintain sufficient cerebral blood flow to sustain consciousness.

Another characteristic of the wounded man, described by many investigators, is thirst. Thirst seems to be a characteristic of the injured person and is found in most emergency room patients brought in acutely ill from trauma with or without shock. The studies carried out to elucidate the nature of the thirst are many and varied. Most of these patients have intense adrenal medullary stimulation from trauma, not necessarily accompanied by shock. Consequently caution must be used in allowing water, since dangerous water intoxication may be induced by this intense stimulus to imbibe liquids in the face of altered renal function.

Another characteristic of the patient in hemorrhagic shock is the low peripheral venous pressure, which is manifest by empty peripheral veins on inspection. Indeed, the starting of a simple intravenous infusion in a patient in hemorrhagic shock can be quite difficult. Obviously there are exceptions, such as shock due to cardiac tamponade, in which there is restriction to inflow of blood to the right side of the heart. In this instance the peripheral veins, including the neck veins, will be distended.

Nausea and vomiting from hypovolemic shock are common. It is true that other causes should be sought for, but shock alone may be first manifest in this manner.

Another classic finding in hemorrhagic hypovolemia is a fall in body "core" temperature. Whether this is due to a lowered metabolic rate or to lower perfusion in areas where body temperature is measured is debatable.

PHYSIOLOGIC CHANGES

Blood Pressure

Arterial blood pressure is normally maintained by the cardiac output and the peripheral vascular resistance. Thus, when the cardiac output is reduced because of loss of intravascular volume, the blood pressure may remain normal so long as the total peripheral vascular resistance can be increased to compensate for the reduction in cardiac output. The vascular resistance varies for different organs and in different parts of the same organ, depending on the local conditions that determine the state of vasoconstriction or vasodilatation at the time of the loss of intravascular volume. An example of the differential increase in peripheral resistance with reduction in cardiac output is seen in the change in distributional total blood flow to organs such as the heart and the brain as opposed to that to most other organs which are not essential for immediate survival. In hemorrhagic shock the heart may receive 25 per cent of the total cardiac output as opposed to the normal 5 to 8 per cent. The great increase in peripheral resistance in such organs as the skin and the kidney causes significant reduction in flow in these organs while providing a lifesaving diversion of the cardiac output to the brain and the heart.

Consequently the blood pressure may not fall until the reduction in cardiac output or loss of blood volume is so great that the adaptive homeostatic mechanisms can no longer compensate for the reduced volume. As the deficit continues, however, there is a progressive hypotension.

Pulse Rate

Characteristically, reduction of the volume in the vascular tree is associated with tachycardia. A fall in pressure within the great vessels results in excitation of the sympathico-adrenal division of the autonomic nervous system and, simultaneously, inhibition of the vagal-medullary center. Consequently, with hemorrhage or loss of circulating blood volume, the resulting fall in arterial blood pressure should cause an increase in heart rate.

However, this compensatory mechanism is variable in its effectiveness. Obviously, the degree of loss of intravascular volume, the amount of reduction in venous return, and other variables such as ventricular function may markedly influence the ability of Marey's phenomenon to compensate for the reduction in blood volume. Work with slow hemorrhage in normal healthy volunteers by Shenkin et al.[13] has shown that, as long as the supine position is maintained, as much as 1000 cc of blood may be lost without significant increase in pulse rate. Similarly, the pacemaker system of the heart within the sinoatrial node is obviously influenced by other stimuli such as fear and anxiety that may also accompany the trauma producing the loss of intravascular volume.

Consequently, during the course of observation and treatment of shock, changes in pulse rate are of value only when followed over an extended period. Change in pulse rate may indicate response to therapy once other external sources that may have changed cardiac rate are diminished or removed.

Vasoconstriction

Increase in peripheral vascular resistance by production of peripheral vasoconstriction rapidly becomes maximal in an effort to compensate for the reduced cardiac output. Vascular resistance can be measured only indirectly in man and in animals. There is good evidence that early disproportionate reduction in vascular resistance in the heart occurs while there is still little change in vascular resistance in many organs. Subsequently, maximal vasoconstriction occurs in the skin, kidneys, liver and, finally, in the brain.[15]

Concomitantly, there is generalized constriction of the veins in response to reduction in intravascular volume. Venoconstriction would be a necessary homeostatic mechanism since over half of the total blood volume may be contained within the venous tree.[15]

These vascular responses to hemorrhage are immediate and striking. Within seconds following the onset of hemorrhage there are unequivocal signs of sympathetic and adrenal activation. Serum catecholamine levels show prompt elevation indicative of action of the adrenal medullary function.[17] The adrenal cortical and pituitary hormones also show prompt increase in serum levels following shock. Many of the clinical signs associated with shock are simply signs of response of the sympathetic and adrenal medullary system to the insult sustained by the organism.

Hemodilution

All the responses to reduction of intravascular volume eventually result in decrease in volume flow to tissues, and initiation of compensatory mechanisms directed at correction of the low-flow state. One such compensation is movement of fluid into the circulation, resulting in hemodilution. This fluid is commonly known as extra-vascular extracellular fluid, and it has the composition of plasma, but a lower protein content.

It is now clear, however, that the hematocrit or hemoglobin concentration in shock is simply an index of the balance between the relative loss of whole blood or plasma and gain into the blood system of extravascular extracellular fluid. For example, in hemorrhagic hypovolemia there is generally progressive hemodilution, which increases with the severity of the shock state. Obviously, in this circumstance there has been a greater movement of fluid from the extravascular to the intravascular space with the progression of the shock. This is in contradistinction to shock associated with loss of intravascular volume primarily due to plasma loss. High hematocrit shock may occur with massive losses of plasma and extravascular extracellular fluid, such as is associated with peritonitis, burns, large areas of soft tissue infection, and the crush syndrome.

The mechanism of hemodilution following hemorrhage is probably on the basis of the Starling hypothesis: i.e., the reduction in hydrostatic pressure in the capillaries because of hypotension and arterial and arteriolar vasoconstriction results in a shift of the pressure gradient to favor the passage of fluid from the tissue extracellular space into the intravascular capillary bed.

It is worthy of note that the studies of Carey et al. do not demonstrate a significant reduction in serum protein content in patients following hemorrhagic shock and resuscitation.[5, 6]

BIOCHEMICAL CHANGES

The biochemically measurable changes that occur as a response to the stress invoked by shock fall into three fairly well-defined categories. These are (1) the changes invoked by the pituitary-adrenal response to stress, (2) those changes brought about by a net reduction in organ perfusion imposed by a low rate of blood flow, and (3) those changes brought about by failing function within specific organs.

Pituitary-Adrenal

The immediate effects seen from sympathico-adrenal activity are those associated with high circulating epinephrine levels. Characteristically, these include eosinopenia and lymphocytopenia along with thrombocytopenia. This doubtless represents the laboratory reflection of increased circulating epinephrine that, in itself, can be and has been measured to be elevated, as an early response to shock. These changes are nonspecific and are found early in a patient with shock or severe trauma. These phenomena usually disappear rapidly. Other evidences of the pituitary and hormonal response to shock are seen in the well known stress reaction or metabolic responses so well described by Moore.[12] These include a striking negative nitrogen balance and retention of sodium and water, as well as a notable increase in the excretion of potassium.

Low-Flow State

Those changes incident to the low rate of blood flow during shock are now being better understood. More evidence is accumulating to support the observation that, as a result of a decreased blood flow or low rate of perfusion, there is a reduction in oxygen delivered to the vital organs and, consequently, a mandatory change in metabolism from aerobic to anaerobic. In the switch from aerobic to anaerobic metabolism, energy made available by the oxidation of glucose is greatly reduced during shock. The most striking example of a shift in metabolism is the production of an end product, lactic acid, instead of the normal aerobic end product of carbon dioxide. This is reflected in a metabolic acidosis with a reduction in the carbon dioxide combining power of the blood. The available buffer base is progressively decreased by combining with the increased lactic acid, and the respiratory compensation that occurs early in the course of hemorrhagic shock is frequently inadequate. Consequently the progressive decline in pH toward a striking acidosis is thereby hastened. Indeed, in several studies the ability of animals as well as man to recover from shock has been found to correlate rather closely with the degree of lactic acid production and the decrease in the alkali reserve and pH of the blood.

In some cases determination of blood pH may not accurately reflect changes in pH at the cellular level. After the induction of hemorrhagic shock in experimental animals, skeletal muscle surface pH changes precede those in blood, and minimal changes may be masked by the efficient blood buffer systems.[10] Lactate and excess lactate levels correlate well with the clinical impression of the depth of shock, but the injuries producing the shock state have a much greater bearing on ultimate prognosis.[4]

Drucker pointed out that there is a consistent elevation of the blood sugar level in relation to the degree of blood loss and the severity of shock.[7] This was earlier observed in battle casualties studied in World War II and has since been thoroughly confirmed by Simeone and others. It is Drucker's belief that this represents an increase in hepatic glycolysis by the change from aerobic or anaerobic metabolism, while Egdahl believes that there is decreased insulin secretion and decreased peripheral utilization of glucose.[9]

Other evidences of failure of different parameters of cell metabolism have been presented by Thal,[16] Schumer,[14] Mela[11] and Baue.[1]

Organ Failure

The biochemical changes that appear incident to organ failure seem to be dependent in large part on the duration and severity of the shock. The changes in renal function induced by hypovolemia may vary from simple oliguria with a concentrated and acid urine to high-output renal failure with a urine of low specific gravity and high pH, or frank anuric renal failure. Similarly, the blood nonprotein nitrogen content will depend on the degree of impairment in renal function. This may vary from slight to no retention of nitrogenous products to a steep and progressive rise that may require therapy.

Changes in ion concentration, including a rise of serum potassium, are dependent on many things, among them adrenal cortical response, the change in metabolism from aerobic to anaerobic with resultant release of potassium, and also specific changes within tissues invoked by the shock. If renal function is maintained, the rise inevitably seen in serum potassium early after the onset of shock is short-lived, in that the renal excretion of potassium is high during recovery from hemorrhagic shock. If renal function is impaired, the concentration of potassium and magnesium as well as creatine can rise to high levels in the serum.

REFERENCES

1. Baue, A. E., Wurth, M. A., and Sayeed, M. M.: The dynamics of altered ATP-dependent and ATP-yielding cell processes in shock. Surgery, 72:94, 1972.
2. Blalock, A.: Principles of Surgical Care, Shock and Other Problems. St. Louis, C. V. Mosby Company, 1940.
3. Blalock, A.: Shock, further studies with particular reference to effects of hemorrhage. Arch. Surg., 29:837, 1937.
4. Canizaro, P. C., Prager, M. D., and Shires, G. T.: The infusion of Ringer's lactate solution during shock. Amer. J. Surg., 122:494, 1971.
5. Carey, L. C., Lowery, B. D., and Cloutier, C. T.: Treatment of acidosis. Curr. Probl. Surg., January, 1971, p. 37.
6. Cloutier, C. T., Lowery, B. D., and Carey, L. C.: The effect of hemodilutional resuscitation on serum protein levels in humans in hemorrhagic shock. J. Trauma, 9:514, 1969.
7. Drucker, W. R., et al.: Metabolic Aspects of Hemorrhagic Shock: I. Changes in Intermediary Metabolism During Hemorrhage and Repletion of Blood. Surg. Forum, 9:49, 1959.

8. Gross, S. G.: A System of Surgery: Pathological, Diagnostic, Therapeutique and Operative. Philadelphia, Lea & Febiger, 1872.
9. Hiebert, J. M., McCormick, J. M., and Egdahl, R. H.: Direct measurement of insulin secretory rate: Studies of shocked primates and postoperative patients. Ann. Surg., 176:296, 1972.
10. Lemieux, M. D., Smith, R. N., and Couch, N. P.: Surface pH and redox potential of skeletal muscle in graded hemorrhage. Surgery, 65:457, 1969.
11. Mela, L. M., Miller, L. D., and Nicholas, G. G.: Influence of cellular acidosis and altered cation concentrations on shock-induced mitochondrian damage. Surgery, 72:102, 1972.
12. Moore, F. D.: Metabolic Care of the Surgical Patient. Philadelphia, W. B. Saunders Company, 1959.
13. Shenkin, H. A., et al.: On the diagnosis of hemorrhage in man: A study of volunteers bled large amounts. Amer. J. Med. Sci., 208:421, 1944.
14. Shumer, W., Erve, P. R., Obernolte, R. P.: Mechanisms of Steroid Protection in Septic Shock. Surgery, 72:119, 1972.
15. Simeone, F. A.: Shock. In Christopher's Textbook of Surgery. Philadelphia, W. B. Saunders Company, 1964, pp. 58–62.
16. Thal, A. P., and Wilson, R. F.: Shock. Curr. Probl. Surg., September, 1965.
17. Watts, D. T.: Arterial blood epinephrine levels during hemorrhagic hypotension in dogs. Amer. J. Physiol., 184:271, 1956.
18. Wiggers, C. J.: Present status of shock problem. Physiol. Rev., 22:74, 1942.

Pathophysiologic Responses to Shock

Chapter Two

RESPONSE OF THE
EXTRACELLULAR FLUID

EXPERIMENTAL STUDIES

Early Results

Hypovolemic shock is the most common form seen clinically and is also the form that has been studied most intensively both clinically and in the laboratory. Most of our own studies have been carried out using hypovolemic shock produced by external blood loss as the model. A method has been developed which allows the simultaneous measurement of total-body red-cell mass with the use of Cr^{51}-tagged red blood cells; and total body plasma volume with the use of I^{131} and, later, I^{125}-tagged human serum albumin. In addition, total body extracellular fluid can be measured simultaneously with the use of S^{35}-tagged sodium sulfate.[13] These three isotopes are simultaneously injected intravenously, and by the use of appropriate energy-differentiating counting instruments, all three isotopes can be determined after equilibration. Volumes are then determined by the dilution principle using multiple sampling.

In an early study the three spaces were measured; splenectomized dogs were then bled a sublethal, subshock amount of 10 per cent of the measured blood volume. After hemorrhage the three spaces were again measured. The measured loss of red cells and plasma, removed during the hemorrhage, could be detected by the method used. It was shown that the decrease in extracellular fluid volume was only that which was lost as plasma removed during the hemorrhage.[14]

By use of the same model, spaces were measured before and after

15

hemorrhage of 25 per cent of the measured blood volume. This hemorrhage was again sublethal, but did produce hypotension. In this group of animals the loss of red cells and plasma could be measured by the method. In addition, however, the functional extracellular fluid volume as measured by the early S[35]-tagged sodium sulfate space decreased by 18 to 26 per cent of the original volume. Since there was no measurable external loss of S[35] sulfate, this reduction was presumed to be an internal redistribution of extracellular fluid. Subsequent studies of external bleeding of 35 per cent, 45 per cent, and even above 50 per cent hemorrhage always produced the same reduction in functional extracellular fluid, as long as the animal was in shock.

In subsequent studies splenectomized dogs were subjected to "irreversible" hemorrhagic shock according to a modified method of Wiggers, using a reservoir.[16] Return of shed blood in this severe preparation resulted in the return of blood pressure to near control levels followed by a fall in blood pressure within one to 16 hours, with death in 80 per cent of the dogs, a standard mortality rate.

In one group of animals the three volumes were measured; the dogs were then subjected to shock by the Wiggers method. The three spaces were remeasured by reinjection during the period of shock; then shed blood was returned. The decrease in blood volume was that which had been removed. Concurrently, the functional extracellular fluid exhibited a decided reduction. Immediately after the return of shed blood the red-cell mass returned to essentially normal levels, as did the plasma volume; however, there remained a deficit of functional extracellular fluid. In dogs treated with shed blood plus plasma (10 cc per kg) the losses during shock were again similar. After therapy with plasma, plus return of shed blood, there was a return of blood volume to normal. There remained, however, a decrease in functional extracellular fluid volume.

Dogs treated with an extracellular "mimic," such as a balanced salt solution plus shed blood, had comparable losses during shock. As in the previous groups, the blood volume returned essentially to normal after treatment. Dogs treated with salt solution plus shed blood exhibited return of functional extracellular fluid volume to control levels.

In this study only 20 per cent of those treated with shed blood alone survived longer than 24 hours. When plasma was used in addition to whole blood as therapy, 30 per cent of dogs so treated survived. Of the animals treated with lactated Ringer's solution plus shed blood, 70 per cent survived (Fig. 2–1). The 80 per cent mortality of a standard "irreversible" shock preparation was reduced to 30 per cent by restoration of functional extracellular fluid volume in addition to return of shed blood.

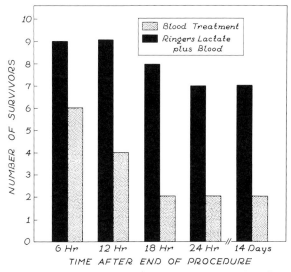

Figure 2–1   Acute hemorrhagic shock—survival study.

All these early studies on the measurement of the functional extracellular fluid were based on volume distribution curves of sulfate measured up to approximately one hour. At any point in the course of the shock volume distribution curve, there will be a reduction in extracellular fluid in the untreated state of shock.

Subsequent work has followed these volume distribution curves out for many hours.[13] In true untreated hemorrhagic shock there is a reduction in the total extracellular fluid, or final diluted volume of radiosulfate, when compared with preshock volumes (Fig. 2–2).

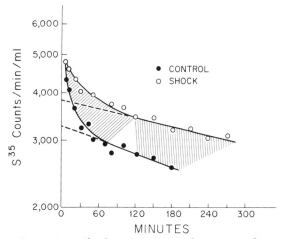

Figure 2–2   Shock—reinjection (splenectomized).

Even when a less severe shock preparation is used, there will still be a reduction in early equilibrating extracellular fluid, or early available extracellular fluid, whereas the total anatomic extracellular fluid may remain normal. Subsequent studies have shown that if shock is not of sufficient duration to produce reduction in both functional and total extracellular fluid, then the reduction may be only in functional extracellular fluid. Furthermore, if therapy is instituted quickly and blood pressure is returned to normal, a long sulfate equilibration curve may fail to reveal the acute reduction which was corrected very early.

Consequently the current status of sulfate as a measure of the functional extracellular fluid must be interpreted in the light that early sulfate space measurement reveals "functional" or "available" extracellular fluid, and that prolonged measurement of these curves will give "total" extracellular fluid values. It must further be remembered that if therapy has been instituted or has been completed, then the "total" or even the "available" extracellular fluid reduction may not be measurable (Fig. 2–3).

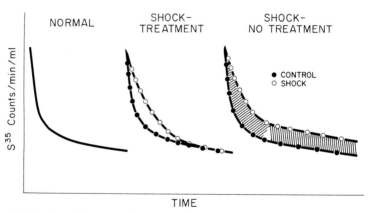

Figure 2–3 Radiosulphate equilibration curve – semilogarithmic plot, summary model.

Recent Cellular Studies

There is no question that some plasma, or transcapillary, refilling does occur in response to hemorrhage and to hemorrhagic shock. This response, however, is initially rather limited and, in severe hemorrhagic shock, is grossly inadequate to explain the reduction seen in interstitial fluid. Since there is no source for external loss, the question arose as to whether interstitial fluid might move into the cell mass in an isotonic fashion (Fig. 2–4).

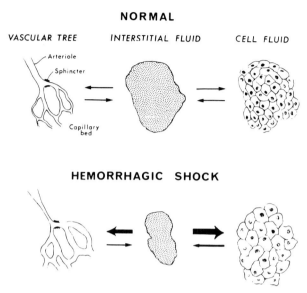

Figure 2–4   Conceptual illustration of interstitial fluid response to hemorrhagic shock.

More recently, studies of ion transport across cell membrane have been undertaken in order to determine the possibility of intracellular swelling in skeletal muscle in response to hemorrhagic shock.[2] By use of a Ling-Gerard Ultramicroelectrode (Fig. 2–5) intracellular transmembrane potential recording has been done with glass-tip diameters of less than 1 micron. This electrode has been modified to record intracellular transmembrane potentials in vivo before, during and after shock (Fig. 2–6).[2]

1. Small Animal Studies. Ling and Gerard in 1949 described a technique that utilizes an ultramicroelectrode to measure directly and accurately the difference in electrical potential between the inside and the outside of a cell.[11] The electrode is made by drawing a piece of borosilicate glass tubing down to a tip less than 1 micron in diameter, and then filling the tube with a buffer solution of potassium salts. The electrode can be inserted transversely through the cell membrane of a muscle fiber without detectable damage to the membrane. The potential of the microelectrode tip, when it is in a buffer solution bathing the muscle, is taken as zero. When the microelectrode is advanced into the surface of the muscle, the potential of the electrode does not change until the tip penetrates a cell membrane. The po-

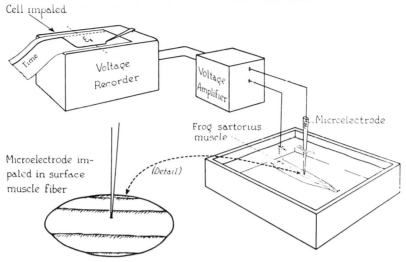

Figure 2–5 Schematic diagram of intracellular recording. (From Woodbury. In: Ruch and Fulton (Eds.): Medical Physiology and Biophysics 18th ed., Philadelphia: W. B. Saunders Company, 1960.)

tential then drops abruptly to −90 mv and remains at this value as long as the electrode remains in the cell. This transmembrane potential is a resting or "steady potential."

With the Ling electrode the system has been modified to record

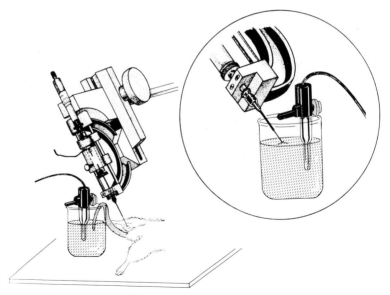

Figure 2–6 In vivo transmembrane potential measurement in rat skeletal muscle.

intracellular transmembrane potentials in vivo (Fig. 2–6).[2] In-vivo measurements in intact animals show consistently reproducible resting membrane potentials in skeletal muscle.

Skeletal muscle transmembrane potentials have been measured in rats and splenectomized dogs by utilizing an in-vivo ultramicroelectrode modified from Ling and Gerard.[2] There was a consistent sustained fall in the transmembrane potential difference (PD) in all animals studied during hemorrhagic shock. The reduction in membrane potential was sustained and not related to changes in concentration of serum potassium, hydrogen, bicarbonate, or carbon dioxide tension. It was, however, related to the shock state.[4]

Subsequent studies outline the use of measurements of PD and analysis of K^+ concentrations in plasma and interstitial fluid in the detection of intracellular and extracellular fluid and electrolyte changes occurring in hemorrhagic shock. The measurements indicate the value of a direct approach to monitoring these alterations and suggest that, in sustained hemorrhagic hypotension, a defective electrolyte transport mechanism exists at both capillary and cell membrane levels.

Baseline and posthemorrhage membrane potential was serially obtained in a manner similar to that previously described, by impalement of individual skeletal muscle cells with standard Ling type electrodes.[2] Electrodes were prepared from borosilicate glass capillary pipets pulled to a tip diameter of approximately 0.2 micron and filled under vacuum with a solution of 2M KCL-0.5M KNO_3. Each electrode was housed inside a thin-bore no. 18 gauge hypodermic needle and mounted on a movable rack and pinion in order to allow percutaneous insertion into the medial muscle mass of the hind limb of the rat (Fig. 2–6). Prior to use, electrodes were connected to the high-impedance side of a circuit through a KCL bridge and balanced to zero potential against a standard calomel electrode on the low-impedance side of the circuit. After muscle penetration the electrode tip was gradually advanced with a micromanipulator so that membrane potential was serially obtained by successive impalement of individual muscle cells.

Interstitial fluid samples were obtained by a modification of the method described by Hagberg and associates in their studies on hemorrhagic shock in dogs.[9] Hydrochloric-acid-cleaned glass pipets with an outside diameter of 1 mm and a 45-degree beveled tip were inserted into a capillary tube holder mounted on a Beckman micromanipulator and connected to a plastic line and syringe for negative-pressure aspiration of samples (Fig. 2–7).

A skin flap was surgically developed on the medial side of the hind limb of the rat in order to expose the connective tissue planes and interstitial compartments surrounding blood vessels and lym-

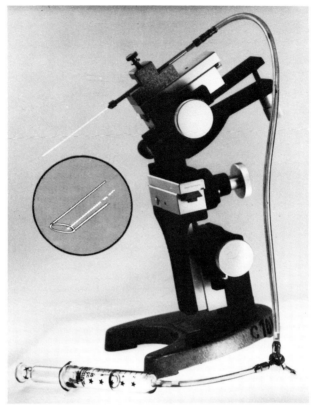

Figure 2-7 Apparatus for microaspiration of interstitial fluid in rat skeletal muscle.

phatic vessels in the femoral area. A continuous drip of water-equilibrated mineral oil was applied to the area of dissection to prevent tissue drying. With the aid of a dissecting microscope, pipet tips were manipulated through the oil layer and into visible interstitial fluid compartments between femoral vessels and muscle groups. Samples of interstitial fluid (40 to 50 nl) were aspirated serially during each experiment (Fig. 2-8). Interstitial fluid samples thus obtained were separated immediately from the admixed oil samples by centrifugation and then transferred to a separate water-equilibrated oil block in another capillary tube for K^+ determination. Matching plasma samples (0.1 to 0.2 cc in volume) were simultaneously obtained from one carotid arterial cannula while blood pressure was recorded from the other.

Care was taken to avoid the rupture of blood and lymphatic vessels surrounding the interstitial fluid compartments. To ensure that no contamination of aspirated samples was occurring, lymphatic

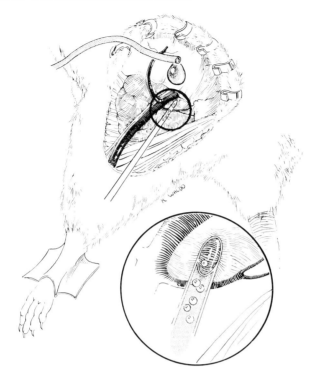

Figure 2–8   Interstitial fluid aspiration in rat hind limb.

radicals in the area of dissection were constantly visualized after injection of 0.5 cc of lisamine green dye into the distal calf muscle of the
animal while Evans blue dye was simultaneously injected arterially
to color plasma. In the presence of both these indicators the interstitial fluid compartments and aspirated samples remained consistently clear and uncontaminated by violation of either vascular or
lymphatic radicals.

The validity of the results of this study is predicated on the
accuracy of the direct measurements obtained for both membrane
potential and extracellular fluid K^+ concentrations. The accurate, direct measurement of the difference in electrical potential between the
inside and outside of a cell has been achieved in numerous labora-
tories since the original descriptions of an ultramicroelectrode by
Ling and Gerard[11] in 1949. Various modifications of the use of this
electrode has allowed in-vivo recording of the resting or "steady state
potential" in both animals and human subjects.[4] The closed percutaneous route of insertion of the small electrode described in this
study has allowed the reproducible recording of membrane po-

tential by successive impalement of single muscle cells without incurring damage to the muscle fibers by the effects of drying or direct trauma. The uniformity of membrane measurements obtained and the similarity to results reported by other investigators indicate stability and reliability of the procedure in the direct assessment of cellular function.

Previous reports from Hagberg and associates have cited the efficiency of a direct approach to obtain interstitial fluid for electrolyte analysis in both control and shock preparations.[9] Securing adequate volumes of interstitial fluid for analysis is much more difficult in shock than in control states, since the presence of well-defined fluid pockets is much less apparent after prolonged hypotension. The consistency with which adequate volumes of interstitial fluid could be obtained during the shock phase of this study is probably due to the continued use of microscopic visualization to locate the sparse volumes of fluid remaining after shock was induced. The similarity of K^+ concentrations in plasma and interstitial fluid samples during control states not only demonstrates that the two compartments are in equilibrium, but also indicates that interstitial fluid samples are not contaminated by K^+ leakage from disrupted muscle cells as long as careful dissection and aspiration techniques are used. The disproportionate rise in interstitial K^+ concentration following prolonged shock appears to be a result of excessive K^+ leakage from muscle cells concomitant with a lack of equilibration between plasma and interstitial compartments resulting from the low-flow state. The presence of elevated interstitial K^+ does not appear to be a result of disruption of muscle cells by the dissection or aspiration technique. Similar elevations were not observed in animals undergoing similar aspiration and dissection, but without sustained shock (Fig. 2–9).[4]

Transmembrane potential difference is generally agreed to be the result of an electrogenic sodium pump or $Na^+ - K^+$ exchange pump with diffusion of Na^+ and K^+ down their respective chemical gradients. Since K^+ permeability is assumed to be much greater than Na^+ permeability in the cell membrane, muscle membrane potential is essentially a K^+ diffusion potential. Although the concentration of K^+ in extracellular fluid rises during prolonged shock, such increases are inadequate to explain the depression of potential which occurs 60 to 70 minutes prior to peak elevations of interstitial fluid K^+. It would appear that the progressive elevation of interstitial fluid K^+ is *preceded* by a fall in membrane potential and results from the combination of continued cellular leakage or a diminished inward transport coupled with a lack of equilibration with the plasma compartment. Since potential is reduced and interstitial K^+ is elevated, there appears to be a great change in the physiologic function of the cell membrane. This change is due to either inhibition of ion pumping or a

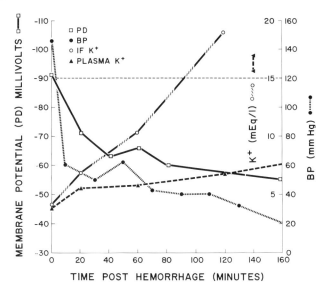

Figure 2–9 Changes in membrane potential and interstitial K⁺ in rats with hemorrhagic shock.

selective increase in membrane permeability to Na⁺. A new balance between active ion pumping and passive cellular leak of ions could result, causing a cellular loss of K⁺ and uptake of Na⁺. As indicated by the Nernst equation, redistribution of passively distributed ions will occur when transmembrane potential is altered by any mechanism. Wilde, in fact, presented evidence that chloride is passively distributed across the muscle cell membrane in accordance with membrane potential.[21] As the level of intracellular chloride increases, Na⁺ will also move inside the cell. The resultant ionic changes would be consistent with cellular swelling.

2. Subhuman Primate Studies. Subsequent studies were performed in baboons to define further the effect of hemorrhagic shock on the ability of the cell membrane to regulate the interchange of materials between the cell and its environment. The "reversibility" of such shock preparations was defined by monitoring changes in cell function following resuscitation. Measurements of PD and an analysis of fluid and electrolytes in skeletal muscle and extracellular fluid were used to assess directly these functional changes. These findings were correlated with data obtained by more classic indirect methods and further delineate the concept of a reversible alteration in membrane transport and are consistent with an in-vivo swelling of skeletal muscle cells in response to severe hemorrhagic shock.

Serial determinations of skeletal muscle PD as well as blood pressure, pulse and respiration were recorded during control and hemorrhagic shock intervals. Arterial blood samples and muscle biopsy specimens for electrolyte and fluid analysis were obtained during the control period and near the end of the shock period, approximately five hours after hemorrhage.

Skeletal muscle membrane potential (PD) was obtained in a manner similar to that previously described by impalement of individual skeletal muscle cells with standard Ling electrodes.[4] Each electrode was housed inside a thin-bore no. 18 hypodermic needle and mounted on a movable rack and pinion to allow percutaneous insertion into the anterior muscle mass of the upper thigh or anterior tibial compartment of the baboon's hind limb (Fig. 2–10). Care was taken to obtain membrane potential recordings from the limb in which no arterial cannulation had been performed. After muscle penetration the electrode tip was gradually advanced with a micromanipulator so that PD was obtained by successive impalement of individual muscle cells. Prior to use, electrodes were connected to the high-impedance side of a circuit through a KCL bridge and balanced to zero potential against a standard calomel electrode on the low-impedance side of the circuit. The tip of the calomel electrode was in electrical contact with the skin of the animal through a potassium phosphate buffer solution ($K^+ - 150$ mEq/L). This was made possible by a plastic cylinder which could be strapped to the anterior surface of the animal's abdomen (Fig. 2–11).

Open biceps brachii muscle biopsies were performed by excising 1.5 to 2.5 gm of lean muscle mass. Opposite extremities were selected for control and posthemorrhage sampling sites. Paired muscle samples

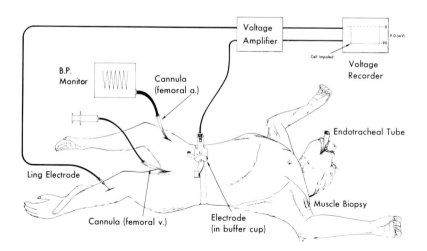

Figure 2–10   In vivo transmembrane potential measurement in primate.

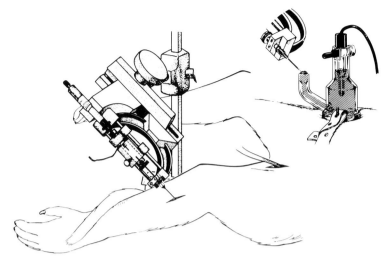

Figure 2–11   Microelectrode holder, manipulating unit, and reference calomel electrode unit in the baboon.

were immediately transferred to tared pyrex tubes, sealed with caps, and placed in a desiccator for two hours prior to determination of wet weight. Utilization of a wet ashing technique rather than a dry method was determined to produce the most complete extraction of muscle electrolytes. Three cubic centimeters of 10 per cent acetic acid were added to one group of wet muscle samples. Muscle electrolytes were leached out by shaking the acetic-acid-suspended wet residues for 72 hours and then autoclaving the samples for 30 minutes (18 psi, 120°C). Sodium and potassium concentrations in serum and muscle extracts were determined by an Instrument Laboratory flame photometer. Chloride concentration was measured by a Cotlove chloridometer. Serum pH, PCO_2 and PO_2 were determined by use of an Astrup gas analyzer. Fat-free dry weight and percentage of water of the matching muscle samples were determined in the following manner: After weighing (wet), samples were dried under vacuum at room temperature for 12 hours and then for 24 hours at 70°C to a constant dry weight. The dried samples were pulverized and fat removed by petroleum-ether extractions. Fat-free dry solid weight was determined after a final period of drying under vacuum at 70°C for 24 hours.

Five animals were additionally studied for purposes of determining the degree of reversibility of the sustained shock preparation described above. After completion of the previously described studies during control and hemorrhagic shock states, resuscitation was carried out by the administration of whole blood and intravenous balanced salt solution. Serial measurements of PD and blood pressure were obtained during initial resuscitation and for several days thereafter. Skeletal muscle biopsies and plasma samples were analyzed for fluid and electrolyte distribution at similar time intervals after resuscitation.

The distribution of water and electrolytes in intracellular and extracellular phases was calculated on the basis of chloride distribution as an estimate of extracellular fluid volume. As predicted by the Nernst equation, the distribution of chloride in intracellular and extracellular compartments was considered to be a passive phenomenon related to the measured resting potential of skeletal muscle.[21] The partition of intracellular and extracellular water and electrolytes was calculated in the following:

$$PD = -61.5 \log. \frac{Cl_o^-}{Cl_i^-} \tag{1}$$

$$Cl_i^- = \frac{Cl_o^-}{\text{Antilog.} \dfrac{PD}{-61.5}} \tag{2}$$

Where:

PD = measured resting potential of skeletal muscle

Cl_o^- = concentration of plasma water chloride

Cl_i^- = concentration of intracellular water chloride (calculated from the Nernst equation)

$$\text{Total sample chloride} = \text{extracellular water chloride} + \text{intracellular water chloride} \tag{2}$$

$$= (ECW)(Cl_o^-) + (ICW)(Cl_i) \tag{2a}$$

$$= (ECW)(Cl_o^-) + (\text{Total sample water} - ECW)(Cl_i^-) \tag{2b}$$

Where:

ECW = extracellular water

ICW = intracellular water

$$\text{Intracellular Na}^+ = \frac{\text{total muscle Na}^+ - (ECW)(Na^+ECW)}{ICW}$$

$$\text{Intracellular K}^+ = \frac{\text{total muscle K}^+ - (ECW)(K^+ECW)}{ICW}$$

The concentrations of Na^+, K^+ and Cl^- in ECW were calculated from their plasma concentrations, correcting for plasma water of 0.94 and the following Donnan factors: Na^+ 0.99, Cl^- 1.01.[19]

Previous studies using muscle biopsy techniques lack the availability of an in-vivo marker to partition extracellular and intracellular distribution of endogenous ions. The use of PD and muscle ion content allows the accurate distributions of ions and water in vivo.

Sustained hemorrhagic shock as previously defined was produced in 22 animals. Figure 2–12 depicts the changes in blood pressure and PD noted to occur in response to sustained hemorrhagic shock in a typical animal (baboon no. 5). The observed parallel between the fall in blood pressure and occurrence of membrane depolarization in response to severe hemorrhagic shock is well established and resembles the relationship described previously in other studies.[4]

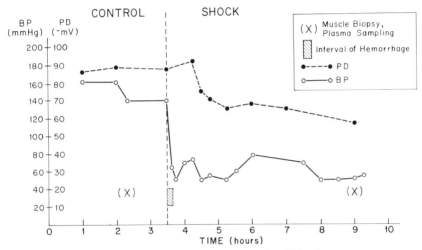

Figure 2-12 Changes in muscle membrane potential and blood pressure in response to hemorrhagic shock.

Table 2–1 compares the average values for resting muscle membrane potential and calculated water partitions in muscle biopsy samples obtained in both control and shock states. PD averaged −90 ± 5.8 mv during the control period. After the onset of sustained hemorrhagic shock, membrane depolarization occurred and PD reached a mean level of −60.9 ± 8.1 mv. Sustained depolarization occurred at an average time of 186 minutes after the onset of hemorrhage and represents a 32 per cent decrease from control levels. Based on calculated chloride distribution at the time of sustained membrane depolarization, there concomitantly occurred a 49 per cent decrease in muscle extracellular water and a 6 per cent increase in muscle intracellular water. As suggested by prior studies, no significant change was noted in the total water content of skeletal muscle samples during prolonged shock despite the above-mentioned redistribution of intracellular and extracellular fluid volumes.[15]

Concomitant with membrane depolarization, hypotension, and a

Table 2–1   Resting Membrane Potential and Water Partition
in Skeletal Muscle During Control and Shock States

	P.D.	TOTAL WATER°	ECW°	ICW°
Preshock	−90.0 mv	0.313	0.037	0.275
	±5.8 mv	±0.016	±0.007	±0.017
Shock	−60.9 mv	0.311	0.019	0.292
	±8.1 mv	±0.017	±0.009	±0.020
% Change	−32%	−0.6%	−49%	+6%

°In 1/100 gm FFDW.

decrease in total or muscle extracellular water in prolonged shock, obvious alterations in plasma and muscle electrolyte concentrations were additionally noted. Table 2–2 summarizes these differences. As expected, serum potassium concentrations increased significantly after prolonged shock (3.1 mEq/L to 6.82 mEq/L) in association with a 10 mEq/L (6 per cent) decrease in intracellular water potassium concentration. Extracellular water concentrations of sodium and chloride did not significantly change after prolonged hypotension.

Sodium concentration in intracellular water increased significantly from control levels of 9.9 mEq/L to shock concentrations of 18.4 mEq/L (+85 per cent). Calculated intracellular chloride increased 185 per cent during the same interval (3.9 mEq/L to 11.1 mEq/L). It is important to note that the internal redistribution of ions following prolonged shock (as depicted in Table 2–2) was not accompanied by a change in *total* electrolyte content of skeletal muscle. Table 2–3 illustrates these values obtained for total electrolyte content in skeletal muscle during control and shock intervals. When expressed as mEq/100 gm of fat-free dry solid weight, the values for sodium, potassium and chloride do not significantly differ in control and shock states.

Table 2–2   Extracellular and Intracellular Electrolyte
Composition During Control and Shock States

	EXTRACELLULAR COMPOSITION (mEq/L)			INTRACELLULAR COMPOSITION (mEq/L)		
	Na^+	K^+	Cl^-	Na^+	K^+	Cl^-
Preshock	146.2	3.1	112.8	9.9	172.6	3.9
	±4.6	±0.4	±3.5	±2.1	±4.8	±0.9
Shock	156.0	6.82	112.1	18.4	162.0	11.1
	±8.3	±3.0	±6.1	±5.0	±12.8	±2.5
% Change	+6%	+118%	−0.6%	+85%	−6%	+185%

Table 2–3   Total Skeletal Muscle Biopsy Electrolyte and
Water Content During Control and Shock States

	Na^*	K^*	Cl^*	H_2O^{**}
Preshock	8.03 ±0.79	47.81 ±2.32	5.19 ±0.64	0.313 ±0.016
Shock	8.40 ±1.33	47.59 ±4.88	5.43 ±0.81	0.311 ±0.017
% Change	+5%	−0.4%	+5%	−0.6%

*mEq/100 gm FFDW.
**1/100 gm FFDW.

In five animals studied after resuscitation from hemorrhagic
shock, the previously mentioned parallel between changes in PD and
blood pressure was again noted. Control PD averaged −92.0±1 mv
and changed to −65.0 ± 3.4 mv after sustained hemorrhagic shock.
Adequate resuscitative efforts produced a reversal of these changes
such that PD returned to normal levels (−89.0 ± 1.0 mv) initially and
remained unchanged during the next several days (Fig. 2–13). As
expected, the changes noted in muscle extracellular water and intracellular sodium concentration in this group of animals were similar to
those in the group previously described. After resuscitation, however,
the abnormalities in intracellular sodium concentration and muscle
extracellular water produced by the hemorrhagic shock process reversed. As illustrated in Figure 2–14, intracellular sodium concentra-

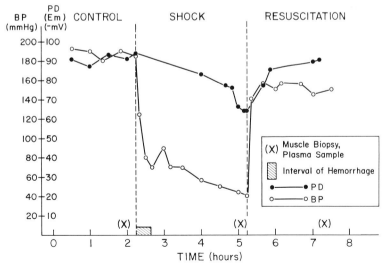

Figure 2–13   Changes in membrane potential and blood pressure during hemorrhagic
shock and after resuscitation.

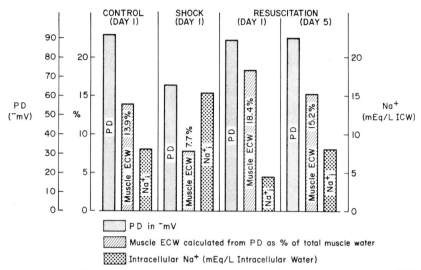

Figure 2-14 Changes in membrane potential, extracellular water and intracellular Na$^+$ after resuscitation from hemorrhagic shock.

tion had risen during the shock period to 15.3 mEq/L, a value almost twice the control. After resuscitative efforts, intracellular sodium concentration fell to extremely low levels (4.36 mEq/L ICW) and over a several day follow-up returned to essentially normal levels. Extracellular water in skeletal muscle decreased significantly during shock in this group of animals, but after resuscitation returned to normal levels and remained so over the next several days.

The data outlined in these experiments confirm the existence of an altered physiologic function of the cell membrane of skeletal muscle cells as a result of the low-flow state produced by severe, prolonged hemorrhagic shock. An assessment of cellular function and composition as well as tissue water partitition in control and shock states was accomplished by use of skeletal muscle transmembrane potential and simultaneous analysis of skeletal muscle biopsy samples.

The skeletal muscle action potentials measured in hemorrhagic shock reveal that amplitude has been decreased approximately 40 per cent (Fig. 2–15). This may be in part due to altered $(Na^+)/(K^+)$ permeability, but it also correlates well with a measured increase in $(Na^+)_i$ from 8.99 mEq/L in the control to 16.1 mEq/l in deep shock. At the same time there was a measured decrease in $(K^+)_i$ from 175 mEq/l in the control to 157.5 mEq/L in shock. Both of these contribute to decreased amplitude and separately can account for the prolonged depolarization and repolarization times.

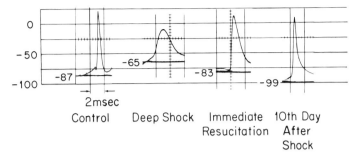

Figure 2–15   Action potentials in primates in hemorrhagic shock.

After resuscitation the membrane recovers slowly. Over 24 hours the depolarization time and amplitude return almost to normal and are normal by the fourth day. Repolarization time, reflecting potassium permeability, $(K^+)_i$ or $(Na^+)_o/(Na^+)_i$, does not return to normal until the tenth day after the shock insult. This would seem to be further evidence that the membrane has incompletely recovered, in that there was a persistent depression of measured $(Na^+)_i$ at 10 days after resuscitation and that muscle extracellular water was expanded. The significance of this incomplete recovery may be important to the total organism and is currently under investigation.

   3. **Interpretation of Experimental Studies.** Concisely stated, reduction in extracellular fluid in reversible hemorrhagic shock can consistently be shown *(a)* with extracellular fluid makers that enter cells slowly or not at all in the shock state; *(b)* reinjection of the extracellular fluid markers is utilized in the shock state; *(c)* extracellular fluid markers or tracers are allowed sufficient time for equilibration; *(d)* shock measurements are obtained while hemorrhagic shock is sustained; and *(e)* if the shock preparation is sufficiently severe and maintained until there is a change in cellular membrane transport.

   The data obtained from prior experiments support the use of transmembrane potential measurements as an accurate indicator of cellular alterations resulting from the low-flow state of hemorrhagic shock. Severe hypotension is associated with a depression of PD which is sustained in the presence of a continued shock state.[17]

   Transmembrane potential difference is generally agreed to be the result of either an electrogenic sodium pump (with active outward extrusion of sodium from muscle cells by a redox system) or a coupled sodium-potassium exchange pump with diffusion of sodium and potassium down their respective chemical gradients.[3, 7, 10] In the latter theory the relative permeabilities of the membrane to the two ions must be considered and the potential interpreted on the basis of the Hodgkins-Katz-Goldman equation in which pNa^+ (relative sodium permeability) is 0.01. Since potassium permeability is assumed to be much greater than sodium permeability in the cell membrane, the PD is essentially a potassium diffusion potential.

The present data suggest, then, that skeletal muscle cells may be a principal site of fluid and electrolyte sequestration after severe, prolonged hemorrhagic shock. Adjunctive studies by Grossman et al. suggest that similar changes in the intracellular mass of neurons in the brain also occur in response to hypovolemic shock.[8] Furthermore, an increase in cellular water content of both cellular and connective tissue components following hemorrhagic shock has been demonstrated by Slonim and Stahl.[18] Fulton has suggested that connective tissue may be the site of some sodium and water sequestration.[6]

The exact mechanism for the production of electrolyte changes as well as the notable diminution in extracellular water which occurs after hemorrhagic shock is not known. It appears that they may well represent a reduction in the efficiency of an active ionic pump mechanism or a selective increase in muscle cell membrane permeability to sodium, or both (Fig. 2–16).

With a reset membrane potential, extracellular fluid electrolyte concentrations are unchanged. Consequently, from the Nernst equation, intracellular Cl^- must rise from 3.5 to 10 mEq, and intracellular Na^+ from 10 to 22 mEq (Fig. 2–17). For transposition of these data to the previously cited measurements in hemorrhagic shock, a model is shown (Fig. 2–18). This model shows a 10 per cent isotonic swelling

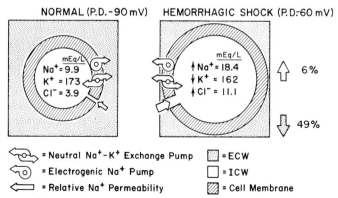

Figure 2–16 Theoretical transport mechanisms responsible for alterations in potential difference (P.D.) and fluid-electrolyte distribution in hemorrhagic shock.

$$E_{Cl} = -61.5 \log_{10} \frac{(Cl^-)_o}{(Cl^-)_i}$$

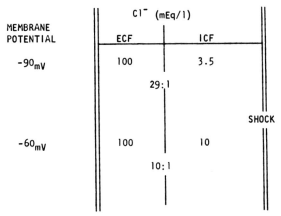

Figure 2–17   Changes in intracellular chloride in response to change in membrane potentials.

of muscle cells to explain the reduction in extracellular fluid measured in hemorrhagic shock. Studies are currently under way to determine the involvement of cell masses other than muscle during the course of hemorrhagic shock.

  4. Other Evidence of Cellular Response.   a. Red blood cells have been studied for further evidence of cellular response to shock.

  Thirty-nine patients in three categories were studied for control purposes (Fig. 2–19). Mean red cell electrolytes (expressed as mEq/L packed red cells) for 24 normal volunteers were 7.5 ± 2.1 mEq of sodium and 96.4 ± 4.0 mEq of potassium.[5] These values compare favor-

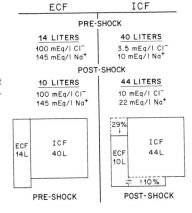

Figure 2–18   Schema of intracellular movement of extracellular electrolytes and water in response to hemorrhagic shock in man.

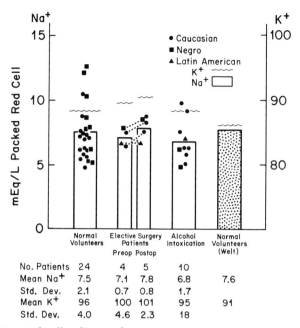

	Normal Volunteers	Elective Surgery Patients Preop	Postop	Alcohol Intoxication	Normal Volunteers (Welt)
No. Patients	24	4	5	10	
Mean Na⁺	7.5	7.1	7.8	6.8	7.6
Std. Dev.	2.1	0.7	0.8	1.7	
Mean K⁺	96	100	101	95	91
Std. Dev.	4.0	4.6	2.3	18	

Figure 2-19   Red cell sodium and potassium concentration in control patients.

ably with the normal values obtained by Welt et al.[20] No significant change was noted after elective surgery in five patients with normal preoperative red cell sodium and potassium levels despite the administration of whole blood. Ten alcohol-intoxicated patients with blood alcohol levels of 0.2 per cent or greater were also found to have normal red cell sodium and potassium. These findings suggest that general surgical procedures, general anesthesia, ethanol intoxication and the administration of whole blood exclusively are not associated with abnormalities in red cell sodium or potassium concentration.

The values for red cell sodium and potassium obtained from studies performed on 75 trauma patients are illustrated in Figure 2–20. Normotensive or mildly hypotensive trauma patients demonstrated no elevation in red cell sodium concentration. Normal levels of red cell sodium were also noted in patients experiencing severe hypotension when sampling was performed during the first one to two hours after the fall of systolic pressure to 70 mm Hg or less. Early sampling of burn patients revealed consistently normal red cell sodium levels regardless of the extent of the burn.

In contrast to the normal values for red cell sodium found in the first four groups of trauma patients, decided elevations were noted in patients experiencing severe sustained hypotension for longer than one to two hours (group 4). All patients in this group had blood pres-

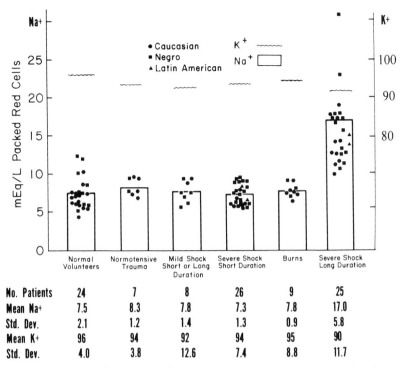

No. Patients	24	7	8	26	9	25
Mean Na+	7.5	8.3	7.8	7.3	7.8	17.0
Std. Dev.	2.1	1.2	1.4	1.3	0.9	5.8
Mean K+	96	94	92	94	95	90
Std. Dev.	4.0	3.8	12.6	7.4	8.8	11.7

Figure 2–20 Red cell sodium and potassium concentrations in normal volunteers, burn patients and hemorrhagic shock victims.

sures less than 70 mm Hg, and the majority had no recordable pressure prior to the institution of resuscitative efforts. Mean red cell sodium concentration in this group of 25 patients increased significantly to 17.0 ± 5.8 mEq/L packed red cells, representing an approximate doubling over values obtained in control patients. Eighteen of these 25 patients were also studied either before the onset of severe prolonged shock or after successful resuscitation (Fig. 2–21). Red cell sodium values averaged 7.6 mEq/L prior to shock and 7.3 mEq/L after resuscitation. As depicted in Figure 2–21, elevation of red cell sodium during hypotensive periods was in strong contrast to the normal values obtained during preshock and postshock intervals in the same subjects. This group of profoundly hypotensive patients thus demonstrated significant elevations in red cell sodium concentration above their separately determined normal values and serve as their own set of controls. A slight decrease in red cell potassium concentration occurred in all groups of trauma patient studies.

When periodic sampling procedures were utilized, sequential changes in red cell sodium concentration were noted in numerous shock victims. Figure 2–22 illustrates the cyclic changes in red cell

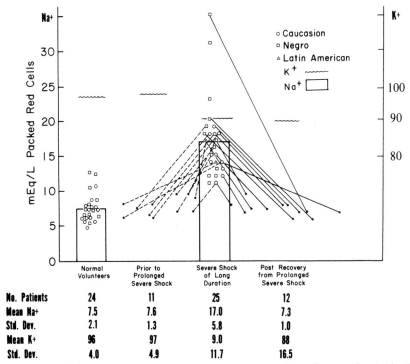

No. Patients	24	11	25	12
Mean Na+	7.5	7.6	17.0	7.3
Std. Dev.	2.1	1.3	5.8	1.0
Mean K+	96	97	9.0	88
Std. Dev.	4.0	4.9	11.7	16.5

Figure 2-21   Sodium and potassium concentrations in prolonged hemorrhagic shock as compared with normal values found in the same patients during control periods.

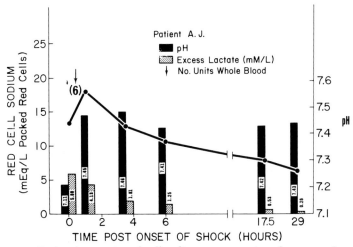

Figure 2-22   Cyclic changes in red cell sodium concentration after onset of reversible shock.

sodium concentration occurring during the resuscitation of a typical patient in prolonged hemorrhagic shock. An elevation of red cell sodium in the range of 12 mEq/L was detected by sampling prior to the institution of resuscitative efforts or the administration of whole blood. Further sodium elevation was noted one hour after resuscitation was begun. After surgery to correct hemorrhage from a lacerated mesenteric artery, the clinical condition of the patient improved and red cell sodium returned quickly to normal levels.

The present study indicates that severe hemorrhagic shock of significant duration is associated with elevation of the internal sodium concentration of the red blood cells. The magnitude of these changes appears to be a function of both the severity and duration of the shock process and seems to correlate well with changes in clinical course when sequential sampling procedures are utilized.

Present data are insufficient to determine the exact cause of the red cell changes observed in profound shock. It can be speculated, however, that the observed elevation in internal sodium concentration in this group of patients is only one manifestation of a process involving a generalized change in cellular composition and function during hemorrhagic shock.

b. Baue has studied cellular function in vitro.[1] He evaluated ATP-dependent and ATP-yielding cell processes in the livers of rats in hemorrhagic shock, before and after treatment. As the metabolic capability of hepatic mitochondria decreased with shock, the cation content of mitochondria was altered and the transport enzyme ($Na^+ - K^+$)-ATPase had greatly increased activity. The cation changes consisted of increased Na^+ and decreased K^+, which could be due to increased Na^+ and K^+ loss from cells during shock and increased Ca^+ and decreased bound Mg. Such cation changes could be responsible in part for the decreased metabolic capability of mitochondria with shock. All these changes were reversible after treatment. This study suggests that alterations in membrane transport may be important causative factors in the initiation of cell injury with shock.

Mela has also studied in-vitro cellular function.[12] Effects of various pH values and increased concentrations of Na^+, K^+ and Ca^{++} ions were evaluated on isolated liver mitochondria in vitro in both the absence and the presence of added bacterial endotoxin and lysosomal enzymes. Low pH and increased Na^+ and Ca^{++} concentrations, in the presence of lysosomal enzymes, were found to be detrimental to mitochondrial function.

Tissue pH was measured in various organs after four to five hours of endotoxemia. The drop in liver pH paralleled the impairment of mitochondrial function and release of lysosomal enzymes. The heart pH, under similar circumstances, increased, as did the heart mitochondrial respiratory activity.

Therefore it is suggested that lowered cell pH and altered cation concentrations, together with lysosomal enzyme release, are damaging to the cellular energy-producing organelles, the mitochondria.

5. Summary. At present it appears that there is a measurable reduction in extravascular extracellular fluid in response to sustained hemorrhagic shock. It also appears that cellular response to hypovolemic hypotension demonstrates a consistent change in active transport of ions. The directly obtained evidence from living cells indicates that sodium and water enter muscle cells with resultant loss of cellular potassium to the extracellular fluid. The interstitial fluid holds the extruded potassium.

Replenishment of the depleted extracellular fluid has been shown to be of significant benefit in the cellular response to hypovolemic shock. It has also been shown to be of clinical benefit in large numbers of patients.

REFERENCES

1. Baue, A. E., Wurth, M. A., and Sayeed, M. M.: The dynamics of altered ATP-dependent and ATP-yielding cell processes in shock. Surgery, 72:94, 1972.
2. Campion, D. S., et al.: The effect of hemorrhagic shock on transmembrane potential. Surgery, 66:1051, 1969.
3. Conway, E. J.: Nature and significance of concentration relations of potassium and sodium ions in skeletal muscle. Physiol. Rev., 37:84, 1957.
4. Cunningham, J. N., Jr., Shires, G. T., and Wagner, Y.: Cellular transport defects in hemorrhagic shock. Surgery, 70:215, 1971.
5. Cunningham, J. N., Jr., Shires, G. T., and Wagner, Y.: Changes in intracellular sodium and potassium content of red blood cells in trauma and shock. Amer. J. Surg., Nov. 1971.
6. Fulton, R. L.: Absorption of sodium and water by collagen during hemorrhagic shock. Am. Surg., 172:861, 1970.
7. Goldman, D. E.: Potential, impedance and rectification in membranes. J. Physiol., 27:37, 1943.
8. Grossman, R.: Intracellular potentials of motor cortex neurons in cerebral ischemia. Electroencephalog. Clin. Neurophysiol., 24:291, 1968.
9. Hagberg, S., Haljamas, H., and Rockert, H.: Shock reactions in skeletal muscle. III: The electrolyte content of tissue fluid and blood plasma before and after induced hemorrhagic shock. Ann. Surg., 168:243, 1968.
10. Hodgkin, A. L., and Katz, B.: The effect of sodium ions on the electrical activity of the giant axon of the squid. *J. Physiol.*, 108:37, 1949.
11. Ling, G., and Gerard, R. W.: The normal membrane potential of frog sartorius fibers. J. Cell. & Comp. Physiol., 34:383, 1949.
12. Mela, L. M., Miller, L. D., and Nicholas, G. G.: Influence of cellular acidosis and altered cation concentrations on shock-induced mitochondrian damage. Surgery, 72:102, 1972.
13. Middleton, E. S., Mathews, R., and Shires, G. T.: Radiosulphate as a measure of the extracellular fluid in acute hemorrhagic shock. Ann. Surg., 170:174, 1969.
14. Shires, G. T., Brown, F. T., Canizaro, P. C., and Somerville, N.: Distributional

changes in extracellular fluid during acute hemorrhagic shock. Surg. Forum, *11*: 115, 1960.

15. Shires, G. T., and Carrico, C. J.: Current status of the shock problem. Curr. Probl. Surg., March, 1966.
16. Shires, G. T., Coln, D., Carrico, C. J., and Lightfoot, S.: Fluid therapy in hemorrhagic shock. Arch. Surg., 88:688, 1964.
17. Shires, G. T., et al.: Alterations in cellular membrane function during hemorrhagic shock in primates. Ann. Surg., *176*:Sept. 1972.
18. Slonim, M., and Stahl, W. M.: Sodium and water content of connective versus cellular tissue following hemorrhage. Surg. Forum, *19*:53, 1968.
19. Van Leeuwen, A. M.: Net cation equivalency (base binding power) of the plasma proteins. Acta. Med. Scand., Suppl., *422*:1964.
20. Welt, L. G., Sachs, J. R., and McManus, T. J.: An ion transport defect in erythrocytes from uremic patients. Trans. Ass. Amer. Phys., 77:169, 1964.
21. Wilde, W. S.: The chloride equilibrium in muscle. Am. J. Physiol., *143*:666, 1945.

Chapter Three

RENAL RESPONSES

The observation was made long ago that during severe shock, from any cause, renal function essentially stops in man. The kidneys, like the skin and the liver, share in the relative oligemia which is a rapid compensatory mechanism in shock to divert blood flow to organs, such as the brain and the heart, most vital for maintaining life. Consequently the relative oligemia suffered by the kidney in response to shock is severe and immediate.

The development of oliguria and, indeed, even anuria is apparently a direct function of the severity and duration of the renal ischemia inevitably attendant on shock. In man, under normothermic conditions, normal kidneys will tolerate renal ischemia for periods varying from 15 minutes to a maximum of approximately 90 minutes.[6] After this degree of ischemia some functional and anatomic changes inevitably occur. With the use of hypothermia, the period of renal ischemia tolerated during hemorrhagic shock can be considerably prolonged,[2] as discussed under Renal Hypothermia, page 130.

SUBCLINICAL RENAL DAMAGE FOLLOWING INJURY AND SHOCK

In civilian and military practice improved resuscitation with balanced electrolyte solution and blood and immediate corrective surgery have resulted in a great reduction in the incidence of primary oliguric renal failure.[3,4] Recognition of nonoliguric renal failure as a less severe form of renal insufficiency suggested that graded renal damage might occur in association with systemic injury. Identifica-

42

tion of patients with subclinical renal damage should be important in their postinjury care.

Patient Studies

A study was undertaken to determine the presence and degree of such renal damage during the early course of severely injured civilian patients. During the period of this study 96,000 patients were treated in the emergency department. Nine hundred eighty-eight of these were admitted to the hospital for care of their injuries. Forty of the most severely injured were selected for continued care in the Trauma Research Unit after resuscitation and operative treatment of injuries.[1] The criteria for inclusion in the present study were hypotension following trauma and multiple long bone fractures. The frequencies of primary bone injury and primary soft tissue injury were approximately equal in the study groups (Table 3–1).

Baseline blood and catheterized urine samples were obtained in the emergency department. Serial six-hour urine collections with midpoint blood samples were obtained from sodium, potassium, urea, creatinine and osmolar clearance during the 72-hour study period.

Glomerular filtration rate (GFR) was measured daily, using inulin or iothalamate I^{125}. Simultaneous para-aminohippurate (PAH) clearances were measured. Clearance substances were administered in 0.9 per cent saline solution by constant infusion pump at rates between 1 and 2 cc/min. A one-hour equilibration period was allowed, after priming, and clearances were measured during a minimum of three 30-minute periods. Saline and air bladder washes through indwelling catheters were done for these clearance determinations. Urine obtained during the inulin, iothalamate-I^{125} and PAH clearance periods was not included in the previously described serial six-hour collections, and appropriate correction for urine minute volume was made during the long clearance periods. All clearances were calculated according to standard formulas. The following indicators were monitored on each patient: direct arterial and central venous pres-

Table 3–1 Renal Function After Trauma

PRIMARY INJURY	
Multiple fractures	21
Aorta or vena cava	7
Other artery	7
Heart	3
Liver	2
	40

sures continuously; intermittent arterial P_{O_2}, P_{CO_2} and pH; and daily blood volume and cardiac output.

All 40 patients showed generalized depression of renal function initially. Within 24 hours of admission, thirty demonstrated return of clearances to normal ranges. The patients were divided into groups according to blood urea nitrogen (BUN) values (Fig. 3–1). Group I, considered to show a characteristic renal response to trauma, was selected on the basis of BUN values continuously below 20 gm per 100 ml after the first hospital day. This group included thirty of the 40 patients. Eight patients with renal dysfunction (group II) showed persistent moderate elevation of BUN values above 20 mg per 100 ml. Two patients showed frank renal failure with rapidly progressing azotemia. One of these patients had sustained a gunshot wound of the renal vein and vena cava and had had the renal pedicle on the involved side clamped for one hour. The other patient, with a gunshot wound of the aortic bifurcation, represented failure of resuscitation. These two patients with renal failure will not be considered in the subsequent comparisons between patients with the characteristic renal response (group I) and those with renal dysfunction (group II). Three patients with direct renal injury requiring suture or partial nephrectomy were included in group I.

As would be expected on the basis of the selection criteria for the groups, GFR was quite different in both groups (Fig. 3–2). Urea clearance (C_{urea}), another clearance primarily related to filtration, was de-

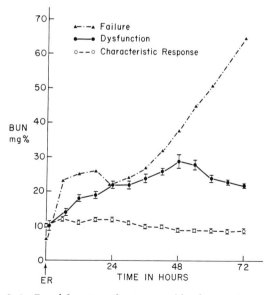

Figure 3–1   Renal function after trauma: blood urea nitrogen values.

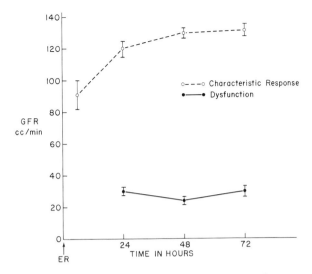

Figure 3–2   Renal function after trauma: glomerular filtration rate.

pressed in both groups initially with a rapid return to and above normal in the characteristic group, and slowly toward normal in the dysfunction group. Urine/plasma (U/P) urea ratio and osmolar clearances (C_{osm}) were different in the two groups only subsequent to 12 hours after admission (Fig. 3–3).

Tubular resorption of water (TcH_2O) was significantly different

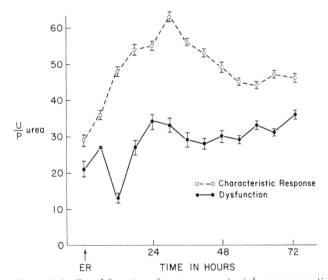

Figure 3–3   Renal function after trauma: urine/plasma-urea ratio.

in the two groups only at 18 and 24 hours after admission. The trend in group I was toward excretion of free water, while the trend in the dysfunction group was toward continued retention of free water. Cardiac output was not significantly different in the two groups (Fig. 3–4).

Sodium clearances (C_{Na}) were similar in the two groups until after 12 hours following admission (Fig. 3–5). Subsequently C_{Na} fell in group II. Postoperative sodium balance, represented as the difference between daily sodium intake and urinary sodium excretion, was different in the two groups. Group I showed positive sodium balance during day 1, balance during day 2 and negative balance during day 3. In group II, the dysfunction group, increasing sodium retention occurred during each of the three days of the study.

There were no discernible differences between the two groups in age, type of injury, length of hypotensive episode, fluid and blood required for resuscitation, postoperative intravenous fluid administration, positive-pressure ventilation, nephrotic antibiotics, minute urine volume, blood volume, or arterial Po_2 and pH.

Discussion

Classic renal clearance techniques have been used infrequently in surgical patients, partly because of errors inherent in the methods.

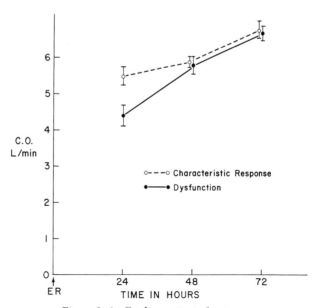

Figure 3–4   Cardiac output after trauma.

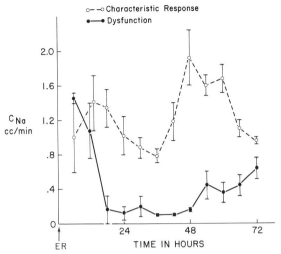

Figure 3–5   Renal function after trauma: sodium clearance.

All renal clearances are urine flow-sensitive. An increase in urine flow leads to a decrease in mean urine transit time. Consequently new filtrate washes out tubular and collecting system contents at a more rapid rate, yielding a factitiously high clearance. Conversely, a decrease in urine flow may lead to a factitiously low clearance. Errors in clearance measurements can be minimized by using constant mechanical infusion, long collection periods and bladder washes. The long collection periods may obscure fluctuations during the period, but provide accurate mean clearances.

In the normal human kidney, glomerular filtration rate may promptly increase 30 per cent above basal level during diuresis.[7, 22] In the above-mentioned study GFR was measured without fluid loading, yet six of the patients in group I showed GFR above 150 cc/min., suggesting the presence of postinjury stimuli in the patients tending to increase GFR maximally. A fall in plasma proteins may be responsible for this observed increase in GFR, since plasma proteins were decreased in the 15 patients in whom measurements were obtained. The patients with renal dysfunction (group II) were presumably subject to similar stimuli, but were unable to respond with any elevation in GFR because of renal damage or persistent nervous or humeral influences affecting GFR.

Endogenous creatinine clearance (C_{cr}) in both groups was always higher than GFR. Notable variation in C_{cr} in the injured patient was noted by Ladd, who concluded that endogenous C_{cr} were unsuitable for evaluation of GFR in battle casualties.[12] Creatinine as determined by the Jaffe reaction overestimates the true creatinine in plasma, and since creatinine is secreted in man, the usual agreement of endogenous C_{cr} with inulin or iothalamate I^{125} clearance is coincidental. Twofold and threefold increases in endogenous C_{cr} occur in association with the changes in muscle metabolism following severe trauma. Apparently normal values for C_{cr} may lead to a false sense of security when, in fact, GFR may be reduced by a factor of two or three in the severely injured patient.

Muscle metabolism is profoundly altered in the injured patient, resulting in increased loads of creatinine and creatine presented to the kidney. In the early postinjury period, group I patients had metabolic changes similar to those found in patients placed on a high protein diet. Even with increases in urea nitrogen load from tissue injury, multiple transfusions and gluconeogenesis, the patients in group I did not undergo azotemia and creatinemia. Only two patients in group I had BUN values as high as 16 mg per 100 ml after the first hospital day, and the remainder had BUN values less than or equal to 11 mg per 100 ml. Azotemia and creatinemia are not inevitable consequences of severe tissue injury, and other factors are operative in the injured patient who exhibits such changes.

Flear and Clark demonstrated that transfused patients lost less nitrogen in the period following injury than similarly injured nontransfused patients.[9] It is not surprising that catabolism and nitrogen excretion are inversely related to the adeqacy of resuscitative therapy. The patients with the greatest catabolic responses had sustained a more severe injury than the patients who did not demonstrate such changes. Flear et al. also demonstrated that transfused patients had negative sodium balances after the first postoperative day as did group I patients in the present study. Whether or not the association of renal dysfunction and sodium retention in group II is a causal one, both seem to result from a more severe injury in the group II patients. The nature of the difference in response in the two groups of patients may lie in individual patient differences or in presently unquantifiable differences in degree of primary injury. The earliest possible restoration of circulating volume with electrolyte solution and blood combined with definitive treatment of injuries should decrease the degree of secondary systemic injury.

TcH_2O differences in the two groups were not striking. Both groups had a TcH_2O of approximately 2 cc/min. during the first hospital day with gradual decrease toward positive free water clearance in group I and continued water retention in group II. Presumably this represents continued high levels of ADH release in group II.[26] In both groups TcH_2O of 2 cc/min. apparently represents a relatively fixed upper limit. This makes available approximately 2500 ml plus 1000 ml of water of metabolism daily. Subtracting the 1500 ml of obligatory daily water loss, a fixed 2000 ml of free water is being added to the metabolic economy daily. Patients in the renal dysfunction group usually had higher serum osmolalities than the patients in group I, suggesting a requirement for additional free water in the group II patients. Positive free water clearances were generally seen in group I only during the third hospital day and perhaps might be looked upon as a sign of recovery. However, patients with the most severely damaged kidneys demonstrate positive free water clearances as do septic patients, so that care must be taken in the interpretation of the finding of positive free water clearances.

Trueta first described arterialization of rabbit renal venous blood secondary to stimuli which led to renal failure when prolonged. From these and other observations he developed a concept of renal arteriovenous shunting as a main factor in the development of post-traumatic renal failure. Recent technical improvements in determining internal intrarenal blood flow support his earlier observations.[15] Padula et al. evaluated the effect of equiosmolar loads of mannitol, glucose, urea or sodium chloride on an isolated dog kidney preparation.[17] The administration of each agent was followed initially by a decrease in renal resistance and an increase in directly measured renal blood flow. The administration of mannitol, glucose or urea alone was followed by a decrease in renal O_2 utilization, while the administration of sodium chloride was followed by an increase in oxygen consumption. An interpretation differing from that of the authors would consider the saline-induced increase in O_2 utilization indicative of internal redistribution of renal blood flow to ischemic cortical areas.

Three patients received furosemide some time during the period of this study. Small transient increases of GFR were apparent after administration of the diuretic in some patients. In view of the demonstrated slow improvement in GFR which occurs after resuscitation and injury repair in group I patients (Fig. 3–2), it is difficult to ascribe increases in GFR during this early hospital period to furosemide. None of the group II patients showed significant increases in GFR after administration of furosemide. Further study of changes in GFR after administration of furosemide is indicated, however, in view of reports suggesting a beneficial effect of furosemide on renal function.[19, 20]

C_{urea}, C_{cr}, C_{osm}, U/P urea ratio, U/P creatinine and U/P osmolality ratios have each been proposed as good clinical determinants of renal damage. Objections to the use of creatinine determinations alone have been noted above. Otherwise there is little to recommend any one of these tests over the others, since all relate filtration to some aspect of tubular function. Recognition of the need to measure at least one of the foregoing in urine and plasma simultaneously is important. U/P ratios approaching unity and clearances below 10 cc/min. are diagnostic of some form of renal failure. Attempted diuresis with volume replacement and ethacrynic acid or furosemide is indicated early in the course of patients with apparent post-traumatic renal failure.

A spectrum of secondary renal injury exists after severe trauma, varying from oliguric renal failure to transient depression of glomerular filtration and tubular function. Thirty of the patients in the present study showed initial depression of all renal functions measured with return to normal ranges within 24 hours of admission. Eight patients had significant and persistent depressed renal function associated with sodium and water retention.

Tissue trauma and multiple transfusions do not lead to azotemia in the injured patient with normal renal function. Conversely, even minimal persistent elevations of BUN are uniformly associated with significant renal dysfunction and sodium and water retention.

Identification of the more severely injured patient in the early postoperative phase can readily be accomplished by serial evaluation of the renal metabolism of urea or sodium. Identification of such patients should lead to meticulous supportive care, since the general metabolic reserve of the more severely injured patients is diminished and further insults are poorly tolerated.

HIGH-OUTPUT RENAL FAILURE

Post-traumatic acute renal insufficiency is well recognized as a highly lethal complication. The diagnosis is classically based on persistent oliguria and chemical evidence of uremia after stabilization of the circulation. The clinical course is characterized by oliguria of several days' to several weeks' duration, followed by a progressive rise in daily urine volume until both the excretory and concentrating functions of the kidney are gradually restored.

It is less well recognized that renal insufficiency may occur without an observed period of oliguria. This variant of renal insufficiency has been reported infrequently after burns,[11] head injury[23] and soft tissue trauma.[21] The reported cases are characterized by increasing azotemia, while the daily urine volume remains normal or increased. Many of these patients have an apparently inappropriate increase in urine volume, and the term "high-output" renal failure may best describe this entity, despite a theoretical objection.[14] This type of renal failure has not been noted frequently after trauma, nor has the clinical course been described in sufficient detail for recognition or management.

Patient Studies

A report has been presented to describe the clinical course of acute renal failure without oliguria, to emphasize the problems encountered in management, and to suggest renal ischemia as the basic causative mechanism.[4] The original clinical material consisted of nine patients in whom high-output acute renal failure occurred after trauma. The age of the patients ranged from 19 to 50 years, and all were in good health prior to injury. Seven cases were due to gunshot wounds and two to blunt trauma. Each had severe intra-abdominal injury. The number of organs injured per patient averaged 3.8. Resection of the right lobe of the liver was necessary in three patients, splenectomy in four, unilateral nephrectomy in two, and repair of retroperitoneal damage in seven.

After severe abdominal trauma, these patients were in shock an average of 3.5 hours, the individual times varying from one to six hours. The average blood loss was 4.2 L, and average blood replacement 3.6 L. The recorded blood loss was the amount measured at the time of operation. In most patients external bleeding was minimal. In addition to whole blood, they were given an average of 4 L of Ringer's lactate solution per patient prior to and during the operative procedure.

After operation the diagnosis of renal failure was not immediately suspected, since urine volumes were above 30 cc/hr., and few abnormalities were present in the initial values of blood urea nitrogen, potassium, sodium, carbon dioxide-combining power and chlorides obtained on the first postoperative day.

In all cases not involving direct damage to the urinary tract, the urinalysis after operation showed specific gravities between 1.003 and 1.010; pH of 5.5 to 6.5; and urinary sediments containing at most a few RBC/hpf. and an occasional cast. The urine-plasma ratio of urea nitrogen, determined in two patients on the second day, was found to be slightly below 20:1.

The mean values of the daily urinary outputs for these nine patients can be seen in Figure 3–6. On the day of operation the minimum urinary output was 730 cc. This represented the output for less than 12 hours in each case. There was a progressive increase in the mean urine volume for the first six to eight days, reaching a height of 2,350 cc and returning gradually to normal between the sixteenth and seventeenth days. The only low volumes were observed in an 8-year-old child with extensive blunt trauma requiring nephrectomy. The continued high output of 3 L per day after the sixteenth day occurred in only one patient; the BUN in this patient did not return to normal for 37 days. The ranges denoted by the bars show the extremely high outputs in some patients compared to the relatively normal values in others during the period of azotemia. The highest urine volumes were found in patients with the highest evaluations of BUN.

Figure 3–7 shows a progressive rise of the mean blood urea nitrogen during the six to eight days after injury, and a gradual return to

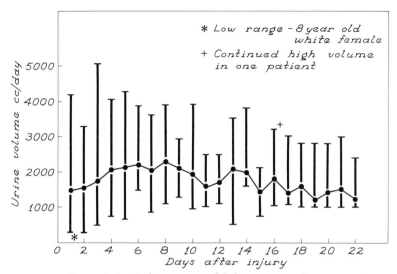

Figure 3–6 High-output renal failure: urine volumes.

normal between the sixteenth and eighteenth days. The serum creatinine levels paralleled the azotemia, the highest value being 6.8 mg
per 100 ml. In all patients the increasing blood urea nitrogen level
was paralleled by an increasing daily urinary volume. Similarly, the
stepwise decline in blood urea was paralleled by a decreasing urinary volume.

In Figure 3–8 the average values and ranges of the serum potas-

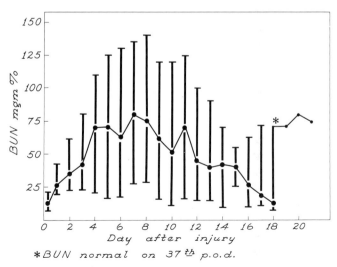

Figure 3–7 High-output renal failure: blood urea nitrogen values.

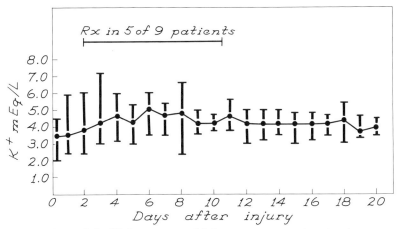

Figure 3–8   High-output renal failure: serum potassium levels.

sium levels are demonstrated. In most instances the initial values after operation were slightly below normal. In five the serum potassium levels were above 6 mEq/L by the second or third postoperative day, while the remaining patients showed a slow but sustained rise. All the accelerated rises resulted from intravenous administration of potassium salts (not more than 60 mEq per day).

When the serum potassium reached 6 mEq/L, treatment with cation exchange resins was instituted. This proved effective in preventing further rises in serum I. In one patient an increase of serum potassium from 5.5 to 9.2 mEq/L was caused by the intravenous administration of 60 mEq of KCl in a 12-hour period. Extracorporeal hemodialysis was necessary to reduce the potassium intoxication that occurred. The bar graph represents the serum potassium levels resulting from the inability of the kidneys to excrete normal amounts of potassium, the administration of potassium salts, as well as the effective use of resins and the artificial kidney.

The mean values and ranges for the carbon dioxide-combining power are seen in Figure 3–9. Moderately low values were present for the first four or five days after injury and represent a mild to moderate metabolic acidosis. All isotonic losses were replaced with lactated Ringer's solution when acidosis persisted. In most patients the acidosis was well controlled by the administration of isotonic lactate solutions, which occasionally resulted in a mild metabolic alkalosis.

Two patients had carbon dioxide-combining power values between 15 and 18 mEq/L despite lactate therapy. These patients died on the tenth and twelfth postoperative days. After the eighth postoperative day carbon dioxide-combining powers were within a normal

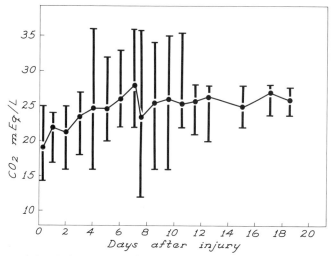

Figure 3–9   High-output renal failure: carbon dioxide-combining power.

range without lactate administration. The serum chlorides did not show a reciprocal relationship to the carbon dioxide-combining powers.

Figure 3–10 presents the average, high and low values for serum sodium determinations throughout the period of renal failure. The highest values of 150 to 154 mEq occurred during a trial of fluid restriction to determine whether the high urinary outputs were being induced by excessive administration of fluids. On these two occasions,

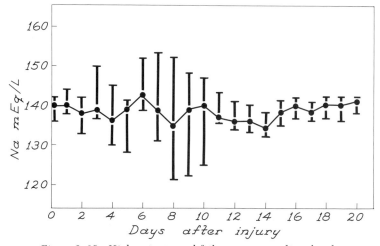

Figure 3–10   High-output renal failure: serum sodium levels.

hypernatremia was readily produced, indicating that the kidney was excreting a solute-poor urine.

Four of the six surviving patients were available for follow-up. Evaluation of renal function was carried out one to $1\frac{1}{2}$ years after injury. Determinations of blood urea nitrogen, creatinine, sodium, potassium, carbon dioxide and chloride were normal. Intravenous pyelography was normal. The lowest urinary concentration (Fishberg) obtained was 1.020, and PSP excretion exceeded 30 per cent in 30 minutes in all patients studied.

Autopsy was performed on the three patients who died. Patient W.B. died on the twelfth postoperative day from gram-negative sepsis, resulting from extensive necrosis of damaged muscle in the abdominal wall, flank and retroperitoneal areas. Patient R.D. expired on the twelfth day from necrosis of remaining liver tissue due to thrombosis of the left hepatic artery. Patient O.C. R. expired on the fifty-second day after injury as a consequence of multiple small bowel fistulas and septic shock (Aerobacter aerogenes blood culture).

Microscopic examination of the kidneys from these three patients showed regenerating patchy tubular necrosis. The damage in each instance was principally to the distal nephron; less severe changes were seen in the proximal segments.

The patient presented below (Fig. 3–11) illustrates a typical course of this variant of renal failure.

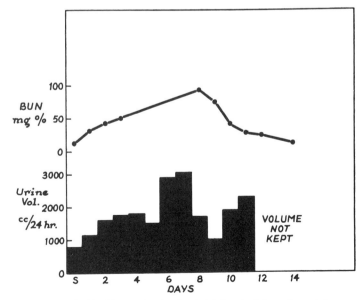

Figure 3–11   Hemorrhagic shock (abdominal hypothermia).

A 24-year-old man was admitted with two 45-caliber bullet wounds in the right upper quadrant of the abdomen. The blood pressure was 40/0 mm. Hg and the pulse rate 150/min. The patient was sweaty, cold, anxious and thirsty, with abdominal rigidity, tenderness, absence of bowel sounds, and minimal distention with flank dullness. A flaccid paralysis of the lower extremities and anesthesia below the twelfth thoracic nerve were present. Roentgenograms revealed a minimal hemothorax of the right chest, one bullet in the tenth thoracic vertebra and another in the left upper quadrant. Hemoglobin was 11 gm per 100 ml. Urinalysis revealed 1+ albumin and an occasional red blood cell in centrifuged sediment. Rapid administration of lactated Ringer's solution (2,000 cc), followed by 1,000 cc of typed (but uncrossmatched) blood produced only transient relief of the shock.

Emergency operation revealed a shattered right lobe of the liver, four perforations of the transverse colon, perforation of both walls of the stomach, and laceration of the lower pole of the spleen and of the upper pole of the left kidney. The right lobe of the liver was resected and splenectomy performed. Suture repair of the stomach, kidney and colon wounds was carried out. A proximal diverting transverse colostomy was performed.

The operative time was 4.5 hours. The measured blood loss was 4,000 cc. Fluid replacement during operation consisted of 3,500 cc of whole blood and 2,500 cc of Ringer's lactate solution. During operation the blood pressure was 70/40 mm Hg except on three occasions when it become unobtainable.

During these intervals the abdomen was sluiced with cold isotonic solution while the larger areas of bleeding were tamponaded. The operation was resumed after 5 to 10 minutes of cooling or when blood pressure was restored. The urine volume measured 890 cc for the 9-hour period from admission until the following morning. After operation the blood pressure was stable at 110/70 mm Hg, pulse rate at 100/min, and the hemoglobin was 10.4 gm per 100 ml.

The graph (Fig. 3–11) records the daily urinary volume and BUN throughout the patient's course. There was a progressive rise in urine volume to 3,200 cc per day on the seventh postoperative day, while the BUN rose steadily to 98 mg per 100 ml.

Forty-eight hours after operation the carbon dioxide-combining power was 19 mEq/L, and the serum potassium was 7.2 mEq/L. The patient had received a total of 60 mEq of potassium chloride in intravenous fluids. Cation exchange resins were begun by rectum, 50 gm every eight hours and continued through the sixth postoperative day, when the serum potassium was 4.5 mEq/L.

The patient received 54 to 81 mEq of sodium bicarbonate (as isotonic sodium lactate) each day for the first six days. The carbon dioxide-combining power ranged between 19 and 22 mEq/L until the seventh day, when a gradual increase began, reaching 28 mEq/L by the tenth day.

This case represents the typical course of high-output renal failure, illustrating the increasing urea nitrogen rise which parallels the increasing urine volume, a mild metabolic acidosis and the acuteness with which hyperkalemia can be produced by the administration of potassium salts. Recognition of the disease entity permitted control of these abnormalities in this patient.

Animal Studies

Animal experiments using dogs were carried out to determine the modifying effect of hypothermia on renal ischemia. After contralateral nephrectomy, the remaining renal pedicle was clamped for two hours in each day.

As seen in Figure 3–12, group A consists of normothermic controls. Group B dogs had regional renal hypothermia produced by irrigation of the peritoneal cavity with cold saline solution. Group C dogs had profound renal hypothermia to 25°C produced by circulating cold saline solution continuously around the kidney. This cooling technique has been previously described.[2]

The results show progressive azotemia and death in untreated animals that are not cooled (group A). There was only transient elevation of the BUN when the kidneys were cooled to 25°C (group C). In group B, regional hypothermia, the BUN rose to an average height of 60 mg per 100 ml by the sixth to tenth day, and gradually returned to normal between the twelfth and sixteenth days.

Utilizing this same model in six dogs with exteriorized ureters, minimum urine volumes of 400 cc per day were obtained without an observed period of oliguria. Usually the daily urine volume increased to between 600 and 900 cc per day before the BUN began to decline. Microscopic examination of these and six similarly treated animals, sacrificed between the fifth and tenth days, showed the tubular lesion to be confined principally to the distal tubules, but with some proximal tubular involvement. These changes, both degenerative and regenerative, were scattered and irregular in distribution.

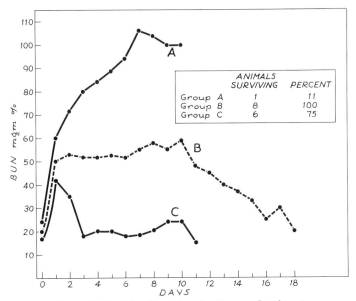

Figure 3–12   Blood urea levels after renal ischemia.

Consequently it can be seen that high-output renal failure in animals is an intermediate form of renal failure. With severe renal ischemia, unmodified oliguric renal failure inevitably resulted. When the kidney was protected with profound hypothermia, no significant renal failure resulted. On the other hand, with modest but practical protection to the kidney afforded by peritoneal sluicing with cold saline solution, moderate elevation of BUN associated with high urine volume was obtained. This protection resulted in recovery of the animal in each instance.

Discussion

Renal insufficiency without oliguria is important from the standpoint of recognition and clinical management of a variant of classic acute renal failure.

The clinical course of patients has been shown to be qualitatively the same as that occurring when oliguria is present. Quantitatively, however, these patients retain a limited ability to excrete acid products of metabolism, potassium and urea. It is of primary importance that renal insufficiency of itself was not sufficient in terms of acidosis, uremia, potassium intoxication or fluid volume control to cause death in this series.

The normal or high daily output of urine, although solute-poor, permits administration of fairly large quantities of water daily, in addition to replacement of isotonic salt losses such as those from gastrointestinal suction. The maintenance of normal extracellular fluid volume and normal serum sodium concentration is, therefore, easily accomplished when accurate daily outputs of each are obtained and losses are replaced accordingly. The quantity of administered fluids containing sodium may be administered as lactate to control the mild metabolic acidosis that occurs. The observations of Moore indicate that if the acidosis is not treated, it may become so severe as to become the outstanding abnormality in these cases.[14]

The chief dangers of high-output renal failure are (1) failure to recognize the existence of renal failure because of normal output and (2) the administration of potassium salts intravenously. Good urinary output and gastrointestinal involvement requiring suction would usually indicate the need for daily replacement of potassium. When this type of renal failure exists, however, potassium intoxication may be produced. In the patients reported here, five of the nine required therapy for hyperkalemia. One of them required emergency hemodialysis for control of excessively high serum potassium levels. It is important that the serum level be determined daily and prior to the administration of any potassium-containing solutions.

The factors involved in the production of acute renal failure following trauma are incompletely understood, but renal ischemia is of unquestioned importance.[6, 8, 10, 18] This concept implies that the ischemia produces damage to the nephrons, which results in failure of the kidneys to excrete urine. Diuresis is felt to represent the recovery phase. Allowing for the physiologic variation between individuals and between given degrees of renal ischemia, a spectrum of the length of the oliguric phase should occur. This has been well documented by Teschan and Mason.[25] Presumably, a few cases of renal insufficiency without oliguria should occur.[13] Although some theorize that renal failure without oliguria should be the most common type of renal failure observed, there is little documented support.[24]

The frequency with which these cases occurred in relation to the small number of oliguric renal failures that were seen during the same period may represent differences in the therapy given during the ischemic episode. There are two outstanding differences in the therapy that we have routinely used. One is the administration of balanced salt solution along with whole blood in the resuscitation from hemorrhagic shock. It has been shown that there is a disproportionate decrease in the extravascular extracellular fluid resulting from severe hemorrhage which results in shock. It is well recognized that prolonged or severe extracellular fluid deficits are necessary for the production of renal failure in animals, and many contribute to renal damage in man.[8] The second difference in treatment is the use of renal hypothermia of a moderate degree to modify or prevent ischemic renal damage. (See Renal Hypothermia, Chapter Six).

Clinical experience and laboratory experiments suggest that high-output renal failure represents the renal response to a less severe or modified episode of renal injury than that required to produce classic oliguric renal failure. Fifty-one such patients have now been documented.

REFERENCES

1. Baker, C. F., Baxter, C. R., and Shires, G. T.: The evaluation of renal function following severe trauma. J. Trauma (in press).
2. Baxter, C. R., Crenshaw, C. A., Lehman, I., and Shires, T.: A practical method of renal hypothermia. J. Trauma, 3:349, 1963.
3. Baxter, C. R., and Maynard, D. R.: Prevention and recognition of surgical renal complications. Clin. Anes., 3:322, 1968.
4. Baxter, C. R., Zedlitz, W. H., and Shires, G. T.: High output acute renal failure complicating traumatic injury. J. Trauma, 4:567, 1964.
5. Brun, C., and Munck, O.: Acute Renal Failure. Inter. Acad. of Path., 82–94, 1966.
6. Defalco, A. J., Mundth, E. D., Brettschneider, L., Jacobson, Y. G., and McClenathan, J. E.: A possible explanation for transplantation anuria. Surg., Gyn. Obst., 120:748, 1965.

7. Doberneck, R. C., Schwartz, F. D., and Barry, K. G.: A comparison of the prophylactic value of 20 per cent mannitol, 4 per cent urea, and 5 per cent dextrose on the effects of renal ischemia. J. Urol., 89:300, 1963.
8. Finckh, E. S.: The failure of experimental renal tubulonecrosis to produce oliguria in the rat. Australasian Ann. Med., 9:283, 1960.
9. Flear, C. T. G., and Clarke, R.: The influence of blood loss and blood transfusion upon changes in the metabolism of water, electrolytes and nitrogen following civilian trauma. Proc. R. Soc. Med., Clin. Sci., 575, 1955.
10. Fudenberg, H., and Allen, F. H., Jr.: Transfusion reactions in absence of demonstrable incompatibility. New Eng. J. Med., 256:1180, 1957.
11. Graber, I. G., and Sevitt, S.: Renal function in burned patients and its relationship to morphological changes. J. Clin. Path., 12:25, 1959.
12. Ladd, M.: Battle Casualties in Korea. U. S. Army Medical Service Graduate School, Walter Reed Army Medical Center, Vol. 4, 1956, pp. 193–233.
13. Meroney, W. H., and Rubini, M. E.: Kidney function during acute tubular necrosis: Clinical studies and theory. Metabolism, 8:1, 1959.
14. Moore, F. D.: Metabolic Care of the Surgical Patient. Philadelphia, W. B. Saunders Company, 1959.
15. Munck, O.: Renal Blood Flow and Oxygen Consumption in Acute Renal Failure Measured by Use of Radioactive ^{85}Krypton. Proc. 1st Int. Cong. Nephrol., Geneve/Evian 1960, pp. 230–235, 1961.
16. Oliver, J., MacDowell, M., and Tracy, A.: The pathogenesis of acute renal failure associated with traumatic and toxic injury. Renal ischemia. Nephrotoxic damage and the ischemuric episode. J. Clin. Invest., 30:1307, 1951.
17. Padula, R. T., Camishion, R. C., Magee, J. H., Noble, P. H., and Cowan, G. S. M.: Evaluation of the protective effect of osmotic diuretics. Adv. in Surg. Res., 1:177, 1969.
18. Phillips, R. A., and Hamilton, P. B.: Effect of 20, 60 and 120 minutes of renal ischemia on glomerular and tubular function. Am. J. Physiol., 152:523, 1948.
19. Powers, S. R.: Maintenance of renal function following massive trauma. Trauma, 10:554, 1970.
20. Powers, S. R.: Renal response to systemic trauma. Amer. J. Surg., 119:603, 1970.
21. Sevitt, S.: Distal tubular necrosis with little or no oliguria. J. Clin. Path., 9:12, 1956.
22. Tanner, G. A., and Selkurt, E. E.: Kidney function in the squirrel monkey before and after hemorrhagic hypotension. Amer. J. Physiol., 219:597, 1970.
23. Taylor, W. H.: Management of acute renal failure following surgical operation and head injury. Lancet, 2:703, 1957.
24. Teschan, P. E., et al.: Post-traumatic renal insufficiency in military casualties. I. Clinical characteristics. Am. J. Med., 18:172, 1955.
25. Teschan, P. E., and Mason, A. D.: Reproducible experimental acute renal failure in rats. Clin. Res., 6:155, 1958.
26. Wright, H. K., and Gann, D. S.: Correction of defect in free water excretion in postoperative patients by extracellular fluid volume expansion. Ann. Surg., 158:70, 1963.

Chapter Four

PULMONARY RESPONSES

Although respiratory failure following injury has recently aroused increased interest, it appears to have been described intermittently since the time of Laennec. The frequency of its clinical occurrence has been obscured by more recognizable and more rapidly lethal problems. Laennec's writings on massive pulmonary collapse contain descriptions of the syndrome we now call post-traumatic pulmonary insufficiency.[53] Deaths from fulminant pneumonia were prominent features in the descriptions of World War I casualties.[16, 27] During World War II Burford described patients suffering pulmonary failure following chest trauma and named this entity traumatic wet lung.[10]

Several recent events have allowed post-traumatic lung failure to gain widespread clinical recognition. Among these were improved management of other problems (e.g. acute renal failure) and the development and clinical application of devices for accurately measuring partial pressures of gases in the blood. In addition, the Viet Nam War with its rapid evacuation and sophisticated resuscitation allowed the emergence of a large "at-risk" population.

In 1968, in response to the rising clinical interest, a symposium on Pulmonary Insufficiency following Nonthoracic Injury was convened under the auspices of the National Science Foundation.[26] The purpose of this meeting was to evaluate the overall incidence of this problem and to attempt to correlate the increasing number of reports from the Viet Nam War of hypoxia following injury with laboratory observations that a variety of insults produced lesions in experimental animals similar to those seen in patients.[38, 50, 80, 84] The compilation of the data from Viet Nam allowed some estimate of the overall incidence of the problem. The largest series presented at this conference indicated that the incidence of isolated pulmonary failure in Viet Nam was approximately 1 per cent of the severely wounded.[62]

CLINICAL PRESENTATION

One of the important products of the 1968 symposium was the synthesis of the clinical picture presented by Dr. Francis Moore and later published in his monograph entitled "Post-Traumatic Pulmonary Insufficiency."[64] He divided the clinical picture into four phases; subsequent observations have further elucidated the meaning and mechanisms of these phases.

Phase 1: Injury, Resuscitation and Alkalosis

This period immediately follows the initial episode of injury, hemorrhage, surgery or sepsis. The patient has been resuscitated by a variety of means, including multiple transfusions, intravenous infusion of balanced salt solutions, antibiotics, anesthetics and surgery, when indicated. With restoration of fluid volume and stabilization of the patient, any initial fixed acid load is oxidized and excreted, and the patient is frequently found to be mildly alkalotic. This alkalosis frequently has a respiratory component due to spontaneous hyperventilation and a metabolic component due to metabolism of transfused citrate and administration of bicarbonate or bicarbonate precursors, such as lactate. Recovery frequently proceeds without event. The likelihood of progressive recovery is indicated by (1) a stable circulatory system, (2) evidence of adequate organ perfusion, including appropriate mentation and normal urinary output, and (3) continued maintenance of effective arterial oxygenation without significant hyperventilation. Signs which portend a less favorable course include (1) cardiovascular instability and the continued necessity for large amounts of blood and fluid, (2) persistently low urine output, (3) other signs of inadequate organ perfusion such as resistant metabolic acidosis, (4) persistent spontaneous hyperventilation, with hypocarbia, and (5) arterial hypoxemia, despite hyperventilation, even in the face of increased inspired oxygen concentrations.

Phase II: Circulatory Stabilization and Beginning Respiratory Difficulty

This period is characterized by apparent stabilization of vital signs and adequate tissue perfusion. Cardiac output continues to be elevated, however, and hyperventilation with significant hypocarbia persists. The arterial PO_2 may be below normal on room air, but partially responds to administration of increased oxygen concentration. The response of arterial PO_2 to an inspired oxygen concentration of 100 per cent, however, falls short of that anticipated. This increase in the alveolo-arterial oxygen gradient on 100 per cent oxygen despite significant hyperventilation with hypocarbia is characteristic of an increased physiologic shunt through the lungs (i.e. perfusion of non-ventilated segments). If the shunted cardiac output is estimated at this time, it may be found to range from 15 to 30 per cent as opposed to the normal shunt fraction of 5 per cent or less. Despite this the patient clinically appears to be doing well.

Phase III: Progressive Pulmonary Insufficiency

In this phase for the first time clinical signs of increasing respiratory difficulty become apparent. The patient becomes dyspneic, his tidal volume continues to increase, and his hypocarbia with hypoxemia become more pronounced. The hypoxemia becomes less responsive to increased concentrations of inspired oxygen. Tidal volumes are frequently large, the spontaneous minute ventilation ranging between 12 and 18 liters per minute. Although the arterial PCO_2 is low, it is higher than would be expected in view of the patient's large tidal volumes. This indicates an increase in dead space ventilation, since large portions of the lung appear to be ventilated without adequate perfusion. At the same time the increased shunt fraction indicates that other areas have continuing or increased perfusion without ventilation.

Endotracheal intubation and mechanical ventilatory assistance are mandatory at this point, but probably should be initiated before the patient reaches this advanced stage. The patient over the next few hours to days may stabilize and begin to improve. Yet even if a patient appears stable, evidence of progression of the pathologic process may be found. The x-ray film, which may have initially appeared normal, begins to show increasing infiltrates and rales, and rhonchi become more evident on physical examination. Markedly increased oxygen concentrations are required to keep the arterial oxygen tension near normal, and the blood pH becomes acidotic.

Infections of various types, particularly associated pulmonary infections, characteristically become more prominent at this stage. Chest x-rays show increasingly widespread areas of consolidation and infiltration, and the strong respiratory drive previously present begins to fade. Eventually the PCO_2 may begin to rise, reflecting increasing dead space ventilation, and increasing efforts are required to support the arterial PO_2.

Phase IV: Terminal Hypoxia and Hypercarbia with Asystole

As the disease progresses, an adequate arterial PO_2 becomes unobtainable, and evidence of inadequate delivery of oxygen to the tis-

Table 4–1   Diagnostic Criteria in Postinjury
Pulmonary Insufficiency

---

1. Major:
   Hypoxemia (unresponsive)
   Stiff lung (low compliance)
   X-ray (diffuse interstitial pattern)
2. Minor:
   ↑ Cardiac output
   Hyperventilation
   Nonthoracic trauma

---

sues with increasing metabolic acidosis occurs. In addition, the
P_{CO_2} may rise above normal. Evidence of inadequate perfusion of
multiple organs becomes manifest by falling urine output, coma and
convulsions. Eventually bradycardia and asystole occur.

Perhaps it is not proper to refer to this as a syndrome, since a
variety of causes may be operative; however, a set of clinical findings
can be described to use for a "diagnosis" (Table 4–1). Most authors
agree that the primary clinical diagnosis is based on (1) the presence
of hypoxia unresponsive to increased inspired oxygen concentrations,
(2) progressively increasing pressure required to achieve adequate
ventilation, and (3) an x-ray picture compatible with diffuse interstitial edema. Minor criteria would include (1) hyperventilation characterized by hypocarbia and (2) an increased cardiac output as much
as two or three times normal. By definition, these patients have some
type of preceding injury, but frequently there is no apparent direct
thoracic injury.

ETIOLOGY

It appears likely that a variety of different injuries can produce a
clinical picture indistinguishable from the one described above.[21] The
most important of these are shown in Table 4–2.

Table 4–2   Etiology of Post-traumatic Respiratory Failure

---

1. Ischemic pulmonary injury	7. Fluid overload
2. Pulmonary infection	Crystalloid
3. Systemic infection (sepsis)	Colloid
4. Aspiration	8. Oxygen toxicity
5. Fat embolism	9. Microatelectasis
6. Microembolism	10. Direct pulmonary injury
Soft tissue Trauma	11. Massive cerebral injury
Multiple transfusions	
Intravascular coagulation	

Hemorrhagic Shock (Ischemic Pulmonary Injury)

The occurrence of pulmonary failure in severely injured patients, many of whom have been in shock, and the demonstration of acute renal failure as a result of renal ischemia led to the assumption that at least part of the respiratory failure following injury might be a result of ischemic injury to the lung. This hypothesis gained support from the early work of Sealy, Webb and several other authors who reported hemorrhage and congestion in canine lungs following hemorrhagic shock and reinfusion of blood.[25, 48, 84, 93] These anatomic changes were similar to those reported in patients by Martin.[58] This hypothesis was widely accepted, and the term "shock lung" was used extensively to describe this clinical syndrome. Retrospective studies from intensive care units implied a correlation between shock and pulmonary failure.[7, 58, 70, 72, 103]

As various investigators began to use hemorrhagic shock as a laboratory model for the study of the mechanism and treatment of post-traumatic pulmonary insufficiency, some question arose as to the relationship between hemorrhagic shock and progressive hypoxia. Even though investigators such as Clowes,[19] Keller,[50] Sykes,[95] Schon[83] and Wilwerth[101] were able to demonstrate gross morphologic changes in dogs, they did not demonstrate a significant defect in oxygenation. With careful blood handling and attempts to prevent atelectasis, a variety of authors have now reported careful studies in dogs, primates and other experimental animals which continue to show anatomic lesions of varying degrees, but do not demonstrate significant or progressive hypoxia.[8, 9, 36, 68] In fact, several studies have shown a decrease rather than an increase in pulmonary shunt fraction during hemorrhagic shock and have demonstrated adequate arterial oxygenation over a period of several days following hemorrhagic shock (Fig. 4–1).[31, 44, 98, 104] A few investigators using extremely severe hemorrhagic shock preparations lasting several hours have been able to demonstrate a preterminal decrease in arterial PO_2 concomitant with generalized circulatory collapse.[51] Even in these studies neither the severity of the clinical syndrome nor its progressive nature has been reduplicated. It should be pointed out that this is in contradistinction to sepsis and septic shock, in which hypoxia has been demonstrated in the laboratory.[34]

Thus, on the basis of laboratory work, it would appear reasonable to question the existence of a direct relationship between hemorrhagic shock and the occurrence of progressive respiratory insufficiency. Despite the absence of conclusive laboratory support, the strong clinical impression of a correlation between hemorrhagic shock and pulmonary insufficiency remains. It is possible that hemorrhagic shock in a laboratory animal cannot produce the same situation which leads to pulmonary failure in patients.

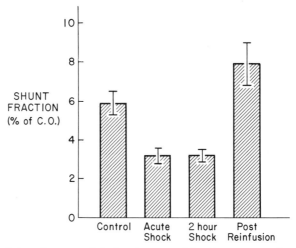

Figure 4–1 Intrapulmonary shunting (measured by the oxygen inhalation method) during and after hemorrhagic shock.

In an attempt to evaluate prospectively the epidemiology of this "syndrome," a series of 49 consecutive patients admitted to the Trauma Research Unit at Parkland Hospital were studied. These patients represented the most severely injured of 978 patients operated upon for injury during this same time period. Thus they represented approximately 5 per cent of the total number of patients admitted to Parkland for injury.

Each of the patients was studied according to the protocol shown in Table 4–3. Determinations were carried out as described on the protocol or more frequently as dictated by the clinical situation. Patients were studied from the time of their admission to the Trauma Unit after operation until the time of discharge from the Trauma Unit or their demise.[46]

For the purpose of data analysis, the patients were divided into four groups according to type of injury. These groups are shown in Table 4–4. Each of the four groups was then subdivided according to the presence or absence of shock. The incidence of pulmonary dysfunction and "classic shock lung" is shown in Table 4–5. Significant pulmonary dysfunction was defined as an arterial PO_2 below 60 mm Hg on room air or comparable hypoxia on increased inspired oxygen concentration. This factor is expressed as a ratio of Pa_{CO_2}/FI_{O_2}, a ratio of less than 300 being considered evidence of severe impairment of ability to oxygenate arterial blood. Classic "shock lung" was defined as defective arterial oxygenation plus evidence of "stiff lung" demonstrated by increasing inspired pressures to maintain tidal volume.[76]

Although arranging the data in this manner makes the number of

Table 4–3 Patient Study Protocol

	DETERMINATION	METHOD	FREQUENCY
Vital signs	Heart rate, respiratory rate	Console monitoring of indwelling catheters	Hourly
	Systolic, diastolic pressure		
	Central venous pressure		
	Pulmonary artery pressure	Swan-Ganz catheter	
	Urine output		
	Intake – IV		
Volume function of lungs	Tidal volume	Wright respirometer or	Every 4 hours
	Minute volume		
	Sigh volume	Ohio 560	
	Effective compliance	calculated from $\dfrac{TV}{IP}$	
	Chest film		Daily
Blood-gas exchange	Arterial and venous		
	PO_2	Radiometer system (Astrup)	Twice daily
	PCO_2		
	pH		
	Cardiac output	Dye dilution	
	FIO_2	IMI O_2 analyzer	
	$A\text{-}VO_2$	Calculated	
	Serum osmolarity		
	Total protein, albumin, globulin	Advanced osmometer	Daily
	Sputum culture		

patients in each group small, several trends are suggested. The greatest incidence of pulmonary dysfunction or "shock lung" is noted in the patients with sepsis *irrespective of the presence or absence of shock.* This apparent correlation is confirmed by comparing all the patients with sepsis to the total group without sepsis (Table 4–6). There is a statistically significant higher incidence of pulmonary dysfunction in patients in the septic group. Furthermore, it would appear that sepsis can produce pulmonary dysfunction without clinical evidence of septic shock.

A similar comparison between the patients in shock and those not

Table 4–4 Patient Groups According to Type of Injury

Group I	– Multiple blunt trauma without thoracic injury
Group II	– Multiple blunt trauma with thoracic injury
Group III	– Sepsis and septic shock
Group IV	– Penetrating soft tissue trauma and/or hemorrhage

A	B
No direct thoracic involvement	Direct thoracic involvement

Table 4–5   Incidence of Pulmonary Failure in 978 Patients

GROUP		TOTAL No.	SIGNIFICANT PULMONARY DYSFUNCTION		"CLASSIC SHOCK LUNG"	
			NUMBER	PER CENT	NUMBER	PER CENT
All patients operated upon for trauma		978	21	2.1	14	1.4
Patients selected for study		49	21	43	14	29
Group I	S	4	0/4	0	0/4	0
	NS	4	2/4	50	2/4	50
Group II	S	5	3/5	60	2/5	40
	NS	8	1/8	12.5	1/8	12.5
Group III	S	5	3/5	60	2/5	40
	NS	5	5/5	100	4/5	80
Group IV A	S	10	4/10	40	1/10	10
	NS	3	1/3	33	0/3	0
Group IV B	S	4	1/4	25	1/4	25
	NS	1	1/1	100	1/1	100

S = Shock.
NS = No shock.

in shock shows no such positive correlation (Table 4–7). In fact, the incidence of pulmonary failure in the patients in shock is somewhat lower than in the remainder of the group. If shock were a prime factor, there would be a higher incidence in the shock group such as that demonstrated in septic patients. The data presented in Table 4–7 include septic patients in both the shock and nonshock group. It is conceivable that the high incidence of pulmonary failure in these patients dilutes the remainder of the data, thus obscuring differences which might occur secondary to hemorrhagic shock. To eliminate this possibility, patients in hemorrhagic shock were compared to patients with-

Table 4–6   Comparison of Septic and Nonseptic Patients

GROUP	TOTAL No.	SIGNIFICANT PULMONARY DYSFUNCTION		"CLASSIC SHOCK LUNG"	
		NUMBER	PER CENT	NUMBER	PER CENT
All patients operated upon for trauma	978	21	2.1	14	1.4
Patients selected for study	49	21	43	14	29
Septic patients	10	8	80	6	60
Nonseptic patients	39	13	33	8	21

Table 4–7   Comparison of Patients with and Without Shock

GROUP	TOTAL No.	SIGNIFICANT PULMO-NARY DYSFUNCTION		"CLASSIC SHOCK LUNG"	
		NUMBER	PER CENT	NUMBER	PER CENT
All patients operated upon for trauma	978	21	2.1	14	1.4
Patients selected for study	49	21	43	14	29
Shock (all types)	28	11	39	6	21
Patients with no shock	21	10	48	8	38

out shock or sepsis. That is, all the septic patients were excluded from both groups. This comparison is shown in Table 4–8. Again (when compared to the patients without shock) there is no correlation between the occurrence of hemorrhagic shock and the incidence of pulmonary failure. It would thus appear that the initial impression of a causative relation between hemorrhagic shock and the occurrence of post-traumatic pulmonary insufficiency is a questionable one. This argument is not intended to deny the existence of pulmonary failure following injury, but to point out a need for changing the emphasis, both on an experimental and a clinical basis. Further efforts to define the origin of this problem seem justified.

Pulmonary Infection

Pulmonary infection is eventually present in virtually all patients succumbing to respiratory insufficiency. This usually becomes clinically apparent during the later stages of the syndrome. Although this

Table 4–8   Comparison of Nonseptic Patients with and Without Hemorrhagic Shock

GROUP	TOTAL No.	SIGNIFICANT PULMO-NARY DYSFUNCTION		"CLASSIC SHOCK LUNG"	
		NUMBER	PER CENT	NUMBER	PER CENT
All patients operated upon for trauma	978	21	2.1	14	1.4
Patients selected for study	49	21	43	14	29
Nonseptic patients	39	13	33	8	21
Patients in hemorrhagic shock	23	8	35	4	18
Patients without hemorrhagic shock	16	5	31	4	25

can certainly compound the syndrome and produce further hypoxia and decreased compliance, it is probably a secondary event and not the initiating cause for the entire clinical picture.[21] There is valid reason for concern about the role of ventilators and other respiratory equipment in the introduction of pulmonary infection. Without proper precautions, devices which are in line with the airway can be a source of bacteria. Pierce and his co-workers have shown that with appropriate measures this can be controlled so that the equipment used for respiratory assistance does not contribute to the incidence of bacterial pneumonia in patients.[73]

Sepsis

Significant extrapulmonary infection with systemic sepsis was a constant finding in our series. By implication, it would appear to be an important causative factor in the occurrence of post-traumatic pulmonary insufficiency. This same finding has occurred in several other clinical series.[11, 21] In fact, Hirsch reported that excluding patients with burns, intracranial lesions and pulmonary contusion, post-traumatic pulmonary insufficiency was rarely seen except in patients with severe sepsis.[43] The concept that sepsis is an important causative agent is supported by a significant amount of laboratory evidence. A variety of septic insults, including injection of E. coli endotoxin, live E. coli organisms, and peritonitis-induced septicemia have been shown to produce both physiologic and anatomic pulmonary derangements.[18, 34, 42] The specific mechanism of pulmonary injury is still speculative, but two factors appear important: (1) There appears to be direct endothelial damage to the pulmonary capillaries with resultant loss of capillary integrity and alveolar injury.[20] (2) Gross disturbances in the clotting mechanism as well as the release of a variety of vasoactive and bronchoconstrictive substances appear to occur with sepsis. This may well result from alteration in the complement system. Whatever the mechanism, there are pronounced changes in vascular resistance and airway resistance plus direct vascular and alveolar injury resulting in interstitial and intra-alveolar edema, hemorrhage, decided changes in surfactants and progressive hypoxia.

Aspiration

Although aspiration of gastric contents is not a universal finding in patients with pulmonary insufficiency, the syndrome produced by severe aspiration with subsequent pneumonia can resemble the clinical picture described above. It would appear likely that in a small but significant number of patients, aspiration (recognized or unrecognized) does occur and may occasionally be the causative factor in production of post-traumatic pulmonary insufficiency.[14, 37]

Fat Embolization

There is little question that the syndrome associated with multiple long bone fractures, which appears to be related to embolization of fat, can produce a clinical picture similar to that described above. There may be mild x-ray differences noted in patients with embolization of fat, although such patients are difficult to separate from the remainder of patients with pulmonary insufficiency following injury.[64] The number of patients in whom significant fat embolization occurs appears to be relatively small. There is considerable evidence, however, that fat embolization may occur unrecognized after significant soft tissue trauma and long bone fractures.[22, 39]

Microembolization

There is a growing body of evidence that microemboli of various sorts with their attendant release of vasoactive substances, injury to pulmonary capillaries and adjacent alveoli and hemodynamic effects can produce defects in pulmonary function. The origin of such emboli and the importance of their role clinically have not been completely elucidated.

One source for such microemboli would appear to be multiple transfusion of stored blood.[65, 94] McNamara and others have shown changes in screen filtration pressure which are presumably due to particulate material in stored blood.[60] The use of dacron wool filters, as described by Schwank, appears to have lowered the incidence of pulmonary problems following extracorporeal circulation. It seems reasonable that such filtration with multiple transfusions would be beneficial. This impression is further supported by the rough correlation between the number of transfusions and the incidence of pulmonary insufficiency following injury in our series as well as in others.[15, 78] This important area certainly requires more exploration. There are several filters available at this time for single unit and multiple transfusions. The efficacy of these filters has yet to be established.

Blaisdell reported an additional source for microembolism.[5] The original publication by Lim and Hall demonstrated embolic material in the venous return following declamping of a cross-clamped aorta.[56] Subsequently, some evidence has been presented indicating that the same kind of embolization may follow massive soft tissue injury, particularly if the extremities have been ischemic for a significant period of time.[91] This is likely operative in an unknown but significant number of injured patients.

A third source of microembolism may be that of disseminated intravascular coagulation. This could result from a combination of massive soft tissue injury, ischemia to the extremities and sepsis with its attendant alterations in the coagulation scheme.

Although it is likely that any or all of these forms of microembolization may be important in the injured patient, their precise mechanism, the diagnosis of such occurrences and specific therapy remain to be established with certainty.

Fluid Overload

The amount of fluids and electrolyte solutions administered to the injured patient has increased significantly over the last several years. This change in therapy is based, in part, on the data and rationale presented elsewhere in this volume. The use of this sort of therapy was applied on a large-scale basis during the Viet Nam conflict. Concomitant with this was an apparent decrease in the incidence of acute renal failure, more efficient cardiovascular resuscitation, and the emergence of respiratory failure as a significant clinical problem. The coincidence of these findings leads to speculation about the role of electrolyte solutions in the production of this syndrome. Some have proposed that in a severely injured patient, one reaches a point at which maintenance of renal function and restoration of adequate organ perfusion in the systemic circulation are gained at the cost of significant fluid overload to the detriment of pulmonary function.[3, 35] Although the definitive answer to this question is not yet apparent, several points are worthy of mention.

First, the effect of massive overload of electrolyte solutions on the cardiovascular system and the lungs has been studied fairly extensively. The study of Terzi and Peters represented evaluation of one of the more extreme overloads.[96] They studied the effects upon anesthetized dogs of the intravenous infusion of balanced electrolyte solutions equivalent to over 30 L in man. They produced fulminant pulmonary edema leading to rapid demise in a significant number of their animals. Yet even under these rather extreme conditions, the animals responded briskly to assisted ventilation and, as long as intermittent positive pressure was employed, did not exhibit hypoxia. Also, the animals which survived this insult appeared to clear their pulmonary edema and did not suffer a progressive disease with hemorrhagic consolidation and the other findings characteristic of the clinical syndrome.

Second, Greenfield in his studies using isolated perfused lungs has evaluated the comparative effects of fluid overload and venous congestion on pulmonary edema and pulmonary function. He also was able to produce pulmonary edema with electrolyte solution overload. Similar to the experience of Peters, this produced only mild hypoxia and not the progressive anatomic lesions described. In contrast, pulmonary edema produced by venous outflow obstruction did produce progressive severe hypoxia and the anatomic findings seen clinically.[33] Thus, although no one would question the fact that massive fluid overload is deleterious to the experimental animals, its role in the production of the syndrome of progressive pulmonary insufficiency remains questionable.

These findings in laboratory animals may not be applicable to patients. In two separate studies from Viet Nam[15, 78] and in the Parkland series there was no correlation between the amounts of fluids received and the development of pulmonary insufficiency.

There is some evidence that the injured lung is more sensitive than the normal lung to fluid overload, and there is general agreement that significant overloads in all patients, particularly in severely injured patients, should be avoided. Nevertheless the role of fluids in the production or compounding of this syndrome remains to be established. Although fluid overload should be avoided, the concept of "drying out" these patients does not necessarily follow as a rational one. Depriving these patients of potentially needed volume may result in inadequate perfusion of kidneys and other vital organs. If the result of excessive fluid restriction is a fall in cardiac output, then the amount of hypoxia resulting from any given amount of pulmonary damage will be compounded.[76] Thus it would appear that the primary answer to fluid therapy at present should be to maintain fluid balance as near normal as possible.

An even more controversial potential cause for this syndrome is colloid administration. It is well established that if the pulmonary vasculature is normal, a fall in the serum oncotic pressure renders the lungs more susceptible to pulmonary edema. One could then reason that if electrolyte solutions are used in the treatment of injured patients, such a fall in oncotic pressure might occur and might be responsible for or compound the pulmonary edema. If this were the case, the administration of colloid might be construed as a potential benefit in these patients. But if the pulmonary capillary membrane is abnormal, the colloids that are administered might be lost into the interstitium, causing an increase in the oncotic pressure of the interstitial fluid and compounding pulmonary edema.[79] The availability of experimental data to resolve these conflicting hypotheses is severely hampered by lack of a reliable experimental model for the syndrome. A variety of reports studying pulmonary capillary permeability and ultrastructure of the pulmonary interstitium have been published.[41, 67, 74, 85, 86, 100] Unfortunately, the majority of these have used hemorrhagic shock as an experimental model and have shown little, if any, change with shock alone. This would lend another small bit of evidence to the concept that hemorrhagic shock is probably unrelated to the disease process at hand. These studies, however, are worthy of mention, since most studies of resuscitation involve blood, fluids and colloid solutions in varying amounts. Some of the studies have shown disruption of the pulmonary interstitial ultrastructure with large amounts of colloid solutions (but little, if any, with large amounts of electrolyte solution), suggesting a deleterious effect of colloid infusion. Nevertheless none of these studies have shown a significant defect in oxygenation with either regimen. One such study conducted in our laboratory is outlined below. The purpose of this study was to establish a method of assessing pulmonary capillary permeability to colloid and to apply it to the problem of capillary integrity in hemorrhagic shock (Fig. 4–2).

Three groups of dogs were studied. Seven control dogs (group I) were injected with 30 μc of dialyzed iodinated I^{125} serum albumin (Risa-125). Plasma samples were taken every 10 minutes for 40 minutes and counted for I^{125}. The dogs were then killed and the lungs rapidly removed and drained of as much blood as possible. Nine biopsies from preselected sites in each lung were taken and counted for I^{125}. The biopsies and whole-lung specimens were weighed wet and then desiccated by vacuum oven for 48 hours to obtain dry weights. Fifteen dogs were given graded doses (100, 200 and 300 mg/kg) of alloxan (group 2) to elicit pulmonary edema varying from minimal to rapidly fulminant prior to Risa-125 studies. Subsequently, 16 dogs were subjected to a two-hour period of hemorrhagic shock (group 3) at a mean blood pressure of 45 mm Hg. Half were allowed to remain in shock an additional two hours, and half were resuscitated with shed blood plus lactated Ringer's solution in a 1:2 volume ratio. Permeability studies were then carried out from one to 72 hours after resuscitation.

The results of all experiments are shown in Table 4–9. Control values were reproducible, as evidenced by the small standard deviations. In the alloxan group the percentage of injected Risa-125 ap-

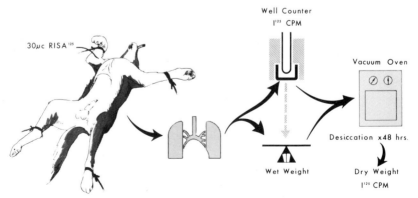

Figure 4–2 Experimental procedure for measuring pulmonary capillary permeability to albumin in animals.

Table 4–9 Lung Colloid Permeability in Hemorrhagic Shock

Group	CPM/GM WET LUNG _____ CPM/ML PLASMA	TOTAL LUNG CPM _____ INJECTED DOSE RISA	DRY WEIGHT _____ × 100 WET WEIGHT
1 Control	0.152 ± 0.03	$2.7\% \pm 0.7$	$21.7\% \pm 0.5$
2 Alloxan			
100 mg/kg...........	0.230 ± 0.07	$4.0\% \pm 1.5$	$20.4\% \pm 1.7$
200 mg/kg...........	0.514 ± 0.15	$17.6\% \pm 8.0$	$15.2\% \pm 2.3$
300 mg/kg...........	0.662 ± 0.04	$24.6\% \pm 4.0$	$15.5\% \pm 0.4$
3 Shock − no reinfusion	0.188 ± 0.02	$3.2\% \pm 1.2$	$22.1\% \pm 0.7$
Shock − reinfusion	0.154 ± 0.03	$2.4\% \pm 0.6$	$20.6\% \pm 0.4$

°CPM = counts per minute of Risa-125; all numbers represent the mean ± standard deviation.

pearing in the lungs varied directly with the amount of alloxan given, ranging from 4.0 per cent ± 1.5 (100 mg/kg) to 24.6 per cent ±4.0 (300 mg/kg). There were no significant changes in dry-wet weight ratios or increased amount of I^{125} leak into the lungs in any shock animals.

The method quantitated fluid and labeled albumin leaks into the lungs when a known increase in pulmonary capillary permeability was induced with alloxan. We concluded from this study that the Risa-125 method is valid and that hemorrhagic shock apparently does not lead to an increased pulmonary capillary permeability to albumin in either treated or untreated animals.[44]

Clinical reports of the use of colloid solutions in the therapy of this syndrome are scanty. The majority involve the use of colloid in conjunction with diuretics.[89] Their beneficial or deleterious effects are difficult to evaluate.

It has been shown that massive overload with colloid-containing solutions can produce pulmonary edema which is more severe than that following overinfusion of electrolyte solutions.[82] Certainly over-infusion with colloid solutions should be avoided, but their role in the induction of this syndrome remains moot.

Oxygen Toxicity

Prolonged use of high oxygen concentrations can result in a clinical picture and pathologic findings similar to those seen in post-traumatic pulmonary insufficiency.[49] The critical levels in healthy patients seem to be between 40 and 50 per cent. There is also a time factor so that the higher the oxygen tension, the less time required to produce symptoms and evidence of damage. The result of this fact has been a conscientious attempt to limit the inspired oxygen concentrations in these patients. Although increased oxygen concentrations may compound the problem late in the course, high oxygen concentrations are not used until the patient has pulmonary problems. It seems extremely unlikely, therefore, that this alone accounts for the syndrome seen. The previous concept of "respirator lung" (direct pulmonary dysfunction induced by ventilatory therapy) appears fallacious. When oxygen concentrations and bacterial contamination are controlled, "respirator lung" no longer occurs.[69, 73]

Microatelectasis

Among the results of immobility, recumbency and sedation is the development of atelectasis. Many of the potential causative factors discused could produce alveolar collapse, and this could account for the hypoxia seen in these patients. It would not explain the apparent increase in dead space ventilation and probably is a result of the insults listed above rather than the primary factor responsible for the clinical picture.

Direct Pulmonary Injury

There seems little question that direct pulmonary injury can produce the progressive syndrome previously outlined. Although most patients considered in this syndrome are thought to have nonpulmonary injury, unrecognized injuries to the lungs may well have occurred.[47] For instance, studies have now shown that a force applied to an animal's abdomen comparable to that of a steering wheel blow received during a head-on collision results in raising the diaphragm to approximately the second intercostal space posteriorly.[71] This may produce a tremendous compressive pulmonary injury which might not be immediately apparent, but may be important in the development of subsequent pulmonary problems

Cerebral Injury

Massive head injury has been associated with acute pulmonary edema, and laboratory evidence of a cause and effect relationship exists.[24, 41, 88] The progression of this acute pulmonary edema to the clinical syndrome under discussion has not been established. Moss has recently proposed that cerebral hypoxia without direct head injury can produce progressive pulmonary insufficiency in animals.[66]

Although the cause of this disease remains unsettled, it seems likely that a variety of injuries can result in a common clinical picture.

More precise definition of the specific causative factors and their mechanisms awaits further investigation. For the present, however, a knowledge of these potential factors can serve as a valuable clinical guide for patients at risk and lead to early institution of therapy when pulmonary failure occurs.

MECHANISM

A review of a basic terminology is shown in Table 4–10.

The hallmarks of this clinical picture are (1) hypoxia which is unresponsive to increased inspired oxygen concentrations, (2) decreased pulmonary compliance (compliance is defined as the amount of volume increase in the lungs obtained by a given change in pressure), which clinically appears as "stiff lungs," and (3) a fall in resting lung volume, specifically a fall in the functional residual capacity.[75, 77] The functional residual capacity as shown in Figure 4–3 is the amount of air remaining in the lungs after a normal expiration.

Hypoxia

The possible causes of hypoxia (decreased arterial PO_2) are shown in Table 4–11. Although all clinicians are familiar with hypoventilation as a cause of hypoxia, such as is seen in the recovery room, it is unlikely that hypoventilation is responsible for the hypoxia in this syndrome. Hypoventilation significant enough to result in hypoxia is associated with a rise in the PCO_2. These patients, however, have abnormally low PCO_2's.

Although diffusion defects can theoretically result from interstitial edema and thickening, diffusion defects should respond to the administration of 100 per cent oxygen. Such is not the case in the patients in question, so that diffusion defects alone would appear to be unlikely causes of the clinical syndrome.

Table 4–10   Basic Terminology and Symbols

$\dot{V}O_2$	Oxygen consumption
C.O.	Cardiac output
$\underline{V}D$	Physiologic dead space ventilation
$\overline{V}T$	as a fraction of tidal volume
Qs/Qt	Venous admixture as a fraction of total cardiac output
A_aD	Alveolar arterial gradient
FI_{O_2}	Fraction of inspired O_2
V/Q	Ratio of ventilation to perfusion

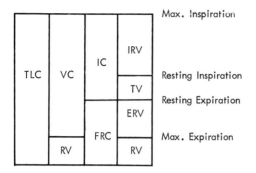

Figure 4–3 Lung volumes and capacities: *TLC*, total lung capacity; *VC*, vital capacity; *IC*, inspiratory capacity; *FRC*, functional residual capacity; *RV*, residual volume; *ERV*, expiratory reserve volume; *TV*, tidal volume; *IRV*, inspiratory reserve volume.

Ventilation perfusion inequalities could explain the hypoxia seen in these patients, and shunting represents the ultimate ventilation perfusion abnormality. This statement deserves further explanation. Normally, there is a balance between ventilation and perfusion within the lung so that a balance exists between ventilation and perfusion of alveolar groups. Compensatory mechanisms exist so that when a group of alveoli become nonventilated or have decreased ventilation, there is a reflex decrease in blood supply to these alveoli. This then results in its extreme in no ventilation and no perfusion to that alveolar unit; thus no abnormality in terms of death space ventilation or shunting occurs.[2, 23] The effects of loss of this normal balance or loss of compensatory mechanisms are shown in Figure 4–4. On the left, alterations in blood flow are demonstrated. It can be seen that progressive decrease in blood flow with continued ventilation affects primarily carbon dioxide elimination. This can be defined as high ventilation to perfusion ratio and is usually reflected by increases in dead space ventilation. Such changes do not result in hypoxia. On the right side of Figure 4–4 is shown the effect of reductions in ventilation while perfusion is maintained. It can be seen that progressive lowering of ventilation can result in hypoxia until the ultimate reduction, i.e., nonventilation, occurs. In theory, as long as any ventilation of the alveolus occurs, the hypoxia should be responsive to oxygen. This then is generally referred to as a ventilation-perfusion abnormality characterized by a low V/Q ratio. When alveolar collapse or nonventilation occurs for any reason, the hypoxia secondary to this is no longer responsive to oxygen, and this is defined as a shunt.

Causes of pulmonary shunting are shown in Figure 4–5. Shunt-

Table 4–11 Causes of Hypoxemia

1. Hypoventilation
2. Diffusion defects
3. V/Q abnormalities
4. Shunting

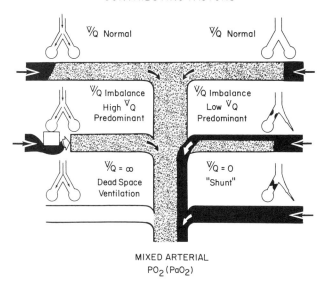

PULMONARY GAS EXCHANGE
CONTRIBUTING FACTORS

Figure 4–4 Diagrammatic representation of ventilation-perfusion ratio ($\dot{V}$/Q) abnormalities.

ing normally takes place to the extent of about 3 per cent of the cardiac output. This is through both intrapulmonary and extrapulmonary routes. Although pathologic shunts occur from extrapulmonary causes, intrapulmonary shunting appears to be the problem in post-traumatic pulmonary insufficiency. Basically, there is perfusion of alveoli which

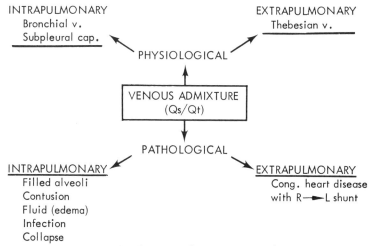

Figure 4–5 Mechanisms of arteriovenous admixture.

are collapsed or for other reasons cannot be ventilated. The alveoli, for example, may be filled with secretions, exudate, blood, edema or protein.

Whatever the cause, the clinical picture appears to result from a distortion of the normal ventilation perfusion balance. This concept is shown in Figure 4–6. In some areas of the lung there appears to be perfusion with poor ventilation, and in other areas there is ventilation of nonperfused alveoli. This would given the consistent findings of decreased resting lung volume (FRC), shunting and increased dead space ventilation.

The concept presented here is simplified, and the entire pathophysiology remains to be elucidated. For instance, intrapulmonary shunting measured by the Xenon method consistently yields a lower shunt fraction than that obtained concomitantly by the oxygen inhalation method.[45] This implies that some areas with very low V/Q ratios which are not atelectatic can act as a "shunt." Studies by other investigators using A-aN$_2$ gradients suggest this same possibility.[57]

For the present, treatment is directed mainly at preventing and controlling hypoxia by supporting lung volume, opening closed alveoli and preventing further loss of functioning lung units.

TREATMENT

In the past, most writings on the treatment of hypovolemic shock stated that breathing high oxygen concentrations is probably of little

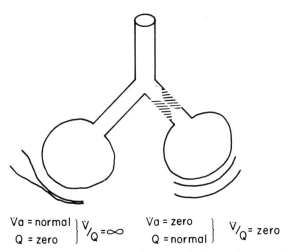

Va = normal
Q = zero $\left.\right\}$ $V/Q = \infty$ Va = zero
Q = normal $\left.\right\}$ $V/Q = $ zero

Figure 4–6   Diagrammatic representation of mismatched ventilation and perfusion.

avail during a period of hypotension.[87] This conclusion was based on the concept that the principal defect is in volume flow to tissues and decreased cardiac output. The oxygen saturation in the majority of patients with uncomplicated hypovolemic shock is generally normal, and the small increase in dissolved oxygen in the blood contributed by raising the P_{O_2} above this level is insignificant, particularly in the face of a markedly decreased cardiac output. This concept continues to be valid in terms of improvement of the shock state or tissue oxygenation. Nevertheless in the small but significant group of patients in hypovolemic shock in whom the oxygen saturation is not normal, the *initial* use of increased oxygen concentrations may be extremely important, since the fall in cardiac output accompanying hemorrhagic shock has been shown to compound existing defects in oxygenation.[76] This may occur in patients with pre-existing defects, such as chronic obstructive lung disease, but more frequently there are problems in oxygenation arising directly from the patient's injury. Examples of this would be a coexisting pneumothorax, pulmonary contusion, aspiration of gastric contents of blood, and larger obstructive problems. Thus, although oxygen is not routinely administered to patients in shock, if any doubt exists as to the possibility of one of these circumstances, or as to the adequacy of oxygenation of arterial blood, the initial administration of oxygen until diligent assessment of the injuries to the patient has been made is certainly justified. Oxygen administered to patients under these circumstances should be delivered through loose-fitting face masks designed for this purpose. If controlled airway is indicated for other reasons, an endotracheal tube is ideal. The use of nasal catheters, particularly those passed in the nasopharynx, is avoided because of potential complications to pharyngeal lacerations and gastric distention. Gastric rupture has been recorded secondary to such a catheter inadvertently placed into the esophagus.

Progressive post-traumatic pulmonary insufficiency usually does not appear during the initial episode of hemorrhagic shock. Although it is likely not a direct result of hemorrhagic shock, this syndrome occurs in the group of injured patients who may have been in hemorrhagic shock.

Diagnostic criteria for post-traumatic pulmonary insufficiency, including those previously given on page 64 are, of necessity, empirical. The institution of therapy, after the classic picture of arterial hypoxia, "stiff lung" and interstitial edema by x-ray has appeared, is unlikely to produce a favorable outcome.[63] The current therapy of this syndrome is largely directed toward prevention of progression (of atelectasis) and support of pulmonary function until the lung can recover from the insult it has sustained.

For this reason, prime consideration is given to identification of

Table 4–12   Patient Evaluation — Monitoring

EKG
Arterial pressure
CVP
Pulmonary artery pressure
Cardiac output
Body weight
Fluid balance
Bacteriologic studies

patients deemed to be in a high-risk group. Such patients are described in the previous section and would include, in particular, patients with massive soft tissue trauma, multiple transfusions, peritoneal contamination, or sepsis. Patients in this high-risk group are
placed in an intensive care unit or similar area where careful evaluation can be made. Most of these patients will have undergone anesthesia and operation and will have an endotracheal tube in place.
When this is so, the endotracheal tube is generally left in place for
several hours until the patient either stabilizes or it is determined that
aggressive pulmonary therapy is indicated. Control of the patient's airway not only makes institution of therapy simpler if indicated, but
also allows more extensive monitoring, as will be pointed out below.

Patient Monitoring

General patient monitoring as listed in Table 4–12 is extremely
important in these patients. In particular, the establishment of an
initial weight for future use in monitoring fluid balance should be
done. Monitoring of pulmonary function can be divided into three
general areas: evaluation of oxygenation, evaluation of ventilation
and evaluation of pulmonary mechanics.

1. Evaluation of Oxygenation.   Clinical and research tools used
for evaluation of oxygenation are shown in Table 4–13. The determination of the partial pressure of oxygen in the arterial blood is the
hallmark of determination of adequacy of oxygenation. But without a
knowledge of the inspired oxygen content, the arterial PO_2 alone is of
minimal use in evaluating pulmonary status.

Table 4–13   Patient Evaluation — Oxygenation

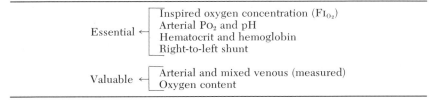

Essential → Inspired oxygen concentration (FI_{O_2})
Arterial PO_2 and pH
Hematocrit and hemoglobin
Right-to-left shunt

Valuable → Arterial and mixed venous (measured)
Oxygen content

Some means of establishing a relationship between the arterial Po_2 and the fraction of inspired oxygen (FIo_2) is essential. The simplest of these is the one used in the Parkland survey, the ratio of arterial Po_2 to FI_{O_2} (Pa_{O_2}/FI_{O_2}). This has the advantage of being immediately applicable at the bedside at any inspired oxygen concentration, and at Po_2's above 60 is fairly reliable. It has the disadvantage that it in no way separates or identifies the cause of the hypoxia. It does not separate hypoxia due to shunting from that due to milder ventilation-perfusion abnormalities or hypoventilation. This is particularly true at low inspired oxygen concentrations. In general, a ratio of 500 is in the normal range and ratios below 300 indicate severe defects in oxygenation. For example, a patient breathing room air ($FI_{O_2} = 0.21$) and with an arterial Po_2 of 60 would have a ratio of 300. A patient receiving 60 per cent oxygen with a Pa_{O_2} of 180 would have an identical ratio.

The calculation of the alveolar arterial oxygen gradient of a patient breathing 100 per cent oxygen for 10 to 15 minutes more nearly points at the cause of the hypoxia and is worthy of discussion. The alveolar oxygen tension in a patient breathing pure oxygen can be obtained by subtracting the vapor pressure of water and the arterial Pco_2 from the barometric pressure. This number can then be calculated and the measured arterial Po_2 subtracted; the resultant difference is the $A-aO_2$ gradient. This measurement suffers from some disadvantage, in that it is somewhat time-consuming and involves subjecting the patient to very high oxygen concentration for a short time. This is not likely to be deleterious to the patient, but may be difficult to achieve in patients who do not have an endotracheal tube in place or other means of airway control. Although the normal $A-aO_2$ gradient is very small, $A-aO_2$ gradients of less than 200 are probably acceptable in postinjury patients. In using these and the remainder of the parameters to be discussed, the trend is more important than the absolute value.

If the fraction of inspired oxygen is held constant, a simpler clinical tool becomes available. Under this circumstances (constant FI_{O_2}) changes in the arterial Po_2 represent changes in the $A-aO_2$ gradient, and changes in the arterial Po_2 alone can be quite useful clinically. In using this method of evaluation, knowledge of the factors which affect the $A-aO_2$ gradient is valuable. These are shown in Table 4–14. Of

Table 4–14   Factors Influencing $AaDo_2$

Magnitude of "shunt"
$A-Vo_2$ difference
Oxygen consumption
Cardiac output
Inspired O_2 concentration
Position of oxyhemoglobin dissociation curve

Table 4–15   Patient Evaluation — Ventilation

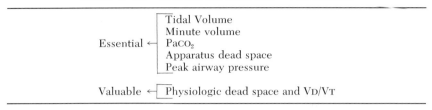

Essential ←	Tidal Volume Minute volume Pa_{CO_2} Apparatus dead space Peak airway pressure
Valuable ←	Physiologic dead space and V_D/V_T

particular importance is the cardiac output. A moderate decrease in cardiac output can result in a fairly dramatic drop in A-aO_2 gradient with no change in degree of pulmonary shunting. In addition, unless the patient is breathing 100 per cent oxygen, change in the arterial P_{O_2} may be the result of hypoventilation.

2. **Assessment of Ventilation** (Table 4–15).   The arterial P_{CO_2} is an extremely useful parameter for the assessment of ventilation. Hypoxia secondary to hypoventilation is uniformly accompanied by an arterial P_{CO_2} greater than normal (above 40). The majority of the patients with post-traumatic pulmonary insufficiency, however, have an arterial P_{CO_2} which is less than normal, and this may be a valuable indicator of potential problems. This is particularly true of a falling arterial P_{CO_2} which is not otherwise explained. Although, in general, measurement of tidal volume requires the presence of either an endotracheal tube or equipment not available in the usual intensive care unit, clinical observations of the rate and depth of patient's respirations can be easily made and are frequently useful indicators of increasing hyperventilation.

3. **Evaluation of Pulmonary Mechanics** (Table 4–16).   Measurement of compliance in postinjury patients is not easily accomplished. There is, however, a fairly close correlation between tachypnea and a fall in compliance. A crude evaluation of the compliance of the lung and chest wall (the effective compliance) can be calculated in patients on a ventilator and used for monitoring.[6] If one divides the tidal volume obtained in a single breath by the change in pressure required to generate that volume, the end result is the effective compliance. This is certainly not proposed as a sophisticated physiologic determination, but has been a useful clinical tool.[46] Its value is enhanced if the breath can be held at the peak of inspiration either voluntarily or by using the ventilator.

4. **Indications for Therapy.**   Our indications for institution of

Table 4–16   Patient Evaluation — Ventilatory Reserve Mechanics

Effective compliance
Functional residual capacity

therapy are shown in Figure 4–7. In general, the therapy given initially is ventilatory support. The particular kind of therapy chosen depends on the clinical situation. The values listed in Figure 4–7 are not absolute and are evaluated according to clinical manifestations. Serial determinations showing changes in the values are much more important than any single determination. For instance, a patient with a Pa_{O_2} of 80 on 40 per cent oxygen who shows no other significant abnormalities probably should not undergo endotracheal intubation and institution of ventilatory support, whereas a patient whose PO_2 progressively fell from 130 to 100 on 40 per cent oxygen over three to four hours should likely be started on some form of therapy.

Worthy of particular emphasis is an alveolar arterial oxygen gradient of over 200. Seventeen of 19 patients evaluated at the Parkland Trauma Unit who failed to raise their PO_2 to 450 on 100 per cent oxygen ($AaDO_2$ greater than 200) eventually required ventilatory therapy. Evidence of unexplained increasing hyperventilation as indicated by a falling PCO_2 or rising minute volume is an indication for institution of therapy.

Ventilatory Support

1. General. Several studies have shown that arterial oxygenation can be improved both in experimental animals and in patients with post-traumatic pulmonary insufficiency by the use of ventilatory support.[12, 55, 81] In addition, improvement in the functional residual capacity can be achieved in this same manner.[77] Initial ventilatory support consists of intermittent positive-pressure breathing employ-

	Acceptable	Institute Therapy
OXYGENATION		
P_aO_2	> 90 mm Hg (40% F_IO_2)	< 90 (40%) or ↓
$Aa DO_2$	50 – 200 mm Hg	> 200 mm Hg or ↑
VENTILATION		
P_aCO_2	35 – 40 mm Hg	< 30 or ↓
Minute Volume	< 12 L/min (?)	↑
MECHANICS		
Rate	12 – 25 / min.	> 25 or ↑
C_{eff}	> 50 cc/cm H_2O	< 50 or ↓

Figure 4–7 Indications for ventilatory support. As discussed in the text, these are not absolute, but are used as general guides. Trends are more important than any single determination.

ing either endotracheal tube or tracheostomy. Tidal volumes of 15 to 20 cc/kg are employed. A significant amount of experimental evidence indicates that higher tidal volumes might be beneficial; however, these are not usually obtainable clinically with safety. The choice between the pressure-cycled and volume-cycled ventilator is an arbitrary one, since theoretically either of these could be used. It has been our experience, however, and that of others that volume-cycled respirators are more satisfactory largely because of their simplicity of use for these purposes and the ability to control more easily inspired oxygen concentration and tidal volume.[75, 77] In addition, patient monitoring is simplified by the use of a volume-cycled ventilator such as the Ohio 560. Initially, then, patients are begun on intermittent positive-pressure breathing using a volume-cycled respirator.

It has now been well documented that under these circumstances greatly increased oxygen concentrations are of minimal benefit in terms of oxygen delivery and are of great potential harm.[75, 77] For this reason every effort is made to keep the inspired oxygen concentrations below 40 per cent. The improvement in oxygenation is obtained by supported ventilation and increasing tidal volume. A partial pressure of oxygen in the arterial blood of 60 to 65 mm Hg is considered satisfactory. Certainly no efforts are made to raise the arterial PO_2 above these levels by increasing the inspired oxygen concentration. This statement is not meant to imply that the level of 60 is normal. Rises above this level *in response to therapy* are considered a favorable prognostic sign. Table 4–17 demonstrates the amount of oxygen which can be carried in arterial blood at a normal hemoglobin and a PO_2 of 65. It can be seen that under these circumstances a patient is carrying as much oxygen in his arterial blood as a postoperative patient with normal lungs and a hemoglobin of 10. Inherent in this concept is the necessity of maintaining the hemoglobin in a range of 12 to 13, attempting to maintain a normal pH, and assuring, as much as possible, that the oxygen-carrying characteristics of the hemoglobin are normal (see Chap. Five).

The success of ventilatory therapy is gauged empirically, and at present only arbitrary guidelines are available. The same monitoring

Table 4–17   Importance of Hemoglobin Concentration in Patients with Pulmonary Insufficiency

Hemoglobin 13.0 — Pa_{O_2} 65 mm Hg
Oxygen content = 16 cc O_2/100 ml blood
Hemoglobin 10.0 — Pa_{O_2} 100 mm Hg
Oxygen content = 13.5 cc O_2/100 ml blood
To reach 16 requires Pa_{O_2} *900*

techniques previously described are used to evaluate the patient's response to therapy. Successful therapy is reflected by a return of these measurements to the acceptable levels previously described. Continued values below those considered in acceptable range or further downward progression of parameters measured are indications for modification of therapy.

2. **Control of PCO_2.** Direct control of the level of the arterial PCO_2 is debatable. Certainly it has been well demonstrated that arterial hypocarbia in and of itself can be deleterious to cerebral circulation and to pulmonary circulation.[32, 61, 92] Consequently, therapy should be constructed so as not to further lower the arterial PCO_2. In general, if the patient is allowed to set his own respiratory rate, increases in tidal volume will be accompanied spontaneously by decreases in rate and no further fall in the PCO_2 will occur. If the patient's respirations are being controlled, then increases in tidal volume must be accompanied by concomitant decreases in respiratory rate, and maintenance of an acceptable level of PCO_2 should not be a problem.

A significant clinical problem occurs because the majority of these patients present with hypocarbia and maintain this in the face of therapy. Some physicians have proposed the use of high carbon dioxide concentrations in the inspired gas and others the addition of dead space to attempt to control the PCO_2.[64, 97] Even with these modalities, control of hypocarbia is extremely difficult to accomplish in the patient who is spontaneously hyperventilating. Dead space can be added to the point of inducing hypoxia in and of itself, and as long as the patient is determining his own respiratory rate, he will continue to increase his rate and to keep his arterial PCO_2 depressed. The same general response occurs when the concentration of carbon dioxide in the inspired gas is increased. Thus effective control of arterial PCO_2 requires heavy sedation or muscle relaxation and control of the patient's respiration. Most are not willing to do this as long as the arterial PCO_2 can be maintained above 30 and no significant uncompensated respiratory alkalosis is present. In patients with the most severe forms of pulmonary dysfunction and severe hypocarbia, respirations must be controlled. Once this decision has been made, a level of arterial PCO_2 between 35 and 40 should be maintained, and this is relatively easy to do.

3. **Constant Positive-Pressure Breathing (CPPB).** More vigorous therapy is required for patients whose disease progresses despite the ventilatory therapy described above. This is particularly true if a satisfactory arterial PO_2 cannot be obtained using IPPB. In our hands, this has consisted in the addition of end expiratory pressure. Ashbaugh and others have shown the benefits of end expiratory pressure (CPPB) in improving oxygenation. Powers has demonstrated increases

in FRC commensurate with the increases in oxygenation.[1, 28, 52, 63] Our usual technique is to begin with 5 to 8 cm of water of end expiratory pressure. Central venous pressure, heart rate, blood pressure, effective compliance and arterial Po_2 are followed closely. If after 15 to 30 minutes no improvement in oxygenation has occurred and no adverse hemodynamic effects have been noted, the end expiratory pressure is increased 2 to 3 cm of water. This is continued in a stepwise fashion until improved oxygenation is achieved or a maximum of approximately 15 cm of water is obtained.

4. Complications.   Ventilatory therapy in general and the use of continuous positive-pressure breathing in particular are not without their complications. Certain precautions are useful in preventing or limiting these complications:

a. The possibility of increased pulmonary infection associated with violation of the airway and nebulizers, and so forth, exists. A study by Pierce at this institution showed an incidence of necrotizing gram-negative pneumonia in autopsy of hospital patients of 1.8 per cent in the pre-IPPB era.[73] This rose to 7.9 per cent in 1963 with the induction of widespread use of ventilatory therapy. By introduction of a vigorous program for the prevention of contamination of nebulizers in ventilation equipment, this incidence was reduced back to its baseline level of 2.1 per cent. This program consisted primarily of cleaning all nebulizers daily with a 0.25 per cent acetic acid solution for 10 minutes. Thus, although infection is a potential significant problem, appropriate care of ventilation therapy equipment would appear to reduce this problem to a minimum level which is present in all extremely ill patients regardless of the use of ventilatory assistance.

b. It is likely that the occurrence of most pneumothorax, pneumomediastinum and other pleural leaks is the result of exceeding safe lung volumes. Although no proved method for avoiding this has been established, there are some guidelines which can be used. In particular, the use of effective compliance for this purpose seems to be beneficial. The overall effect of therapy on effective compliance should be a slow, progressive increase. Certainly, the introduction of increased tidal volume or CPPB should not result in a drop in the effective compliance. On the other hand, as inspiration approaches total lung capacity, the effective compliance does begin to decrease. By use of these concepts the effective compliance can be measured immediately prior to and 15 to 30 minutes after introduction of increases in tidal volume or CPPB. If the change of therapy has resulted in either improvement or no change in the effective compliance, then it is likely within safe limits. On the other hand, if a decrease in effective compliance accompanies increases in tidal volume or an increase in end expiratory pressure, the lung volume may be approaching a dangerous level and the therapy should be cut back to its previous values. By use of this approach the incidence of complications, such as pneumothorax, in patients on CPPB has been reduced from 45 per cent in a previous series to approximately 15 per cent. It is not entirely clear that this drop in complications is due solely to the use of such patient monitoring, since during the same time period the earlier institution of CPPB was employed.

c. A reduction in cardiac output can result from positive pressure ventilation. Some caution is indicated in interpreting falls in cardiac output. As previously stated, the cardiac output in patients with post-traumatic pulmonary insufficiency is frequently elevated. Some of this elevation may be a compensatory change secondary to hypoxia.[63] If satisfactory therapy improves the hypoxia, a fall in cardiac output may represent patient improvement. On the other hand, a fall in cardiac output which results from decreased venous return would produce a further depression of Pa_{O_2}. Such a fall is particularly likely to occur if the patient's intravascular volume is not normal. Patients who have been "dried out" in order to protect their lungs are particularly susceptible to this change. Thus it is our practice to attempt to assure adequate intravascular volume prior to the introduction of respiratory assistance.

When a significant fall in cardiac output occurs as the result of respiratory therapy, a concomitant fall in PO_2 will also occur. Thus arterial PO_2 is measured immediately prior to and following institution of therapy. If Pa_{O_2} is improved or unchanged within 10 to 15 minutes, it is likely that the cardiac output has not been severely impaired. On the other hand, if an abrupt fall in arterial PO_2 occurs after increasing tidal volume or end expired pressure, these should be returned to their previous level and a careful evaluation for the cause of the hypoxia should be made.

d. Frequent auscultation of the chest and chest x-rays are indicated in these patients because of the possibility of pneumothorax and other pleural leaks. The use of prophylactic chest tubes in these patients has been suggested by some and is occasionally made, but this also is not without its complications, and careful physician monitoring is preferable.

Fluid Management

The appropriate fluid management in these patients remains debatable. All agree that blood or fluid overload is to be avoided. Controversy remains whether these patients should be "dried out" or whether fluid balance should be maintained as near normal as possible. The reasons for this disagreement were discussed on page 72. It is our contention that the ideal is the maintenance of normal fluid balance. As has been previously stated, reduction of intravascular volume below normal can compound hypoxia. In addition, hypovolemic patients are more susceptible to abrupt falls in cardiac output with ventilatory therapy.

Careful intake and output records should be maintained. Serial determinations of body weight may provide evidence of undetected changes in fluid status. For example, it has been demonstrated that with the use of efficient nebulizers not only is there a decrease in insensible water loss, but also, in some instances, water can actually be gained through the respiratory tree.[90] A change in the patient's weight is one of the earliest signs of such an accumulation of fluid. Similarly, large unmeasured losses of fluids from dressings and wounds can occur, and, again, a change in the patient's weight is one of the most useful methods for detecting such changes in fluid balance.

Attempts are made to replace only fluids lost and the type lost in these patients in order to maintain normal fluid balance. Albumin is administered in patients who are hypoalbuminemic and show signs of intravascular volume depletion. It is administered in small amounts, very slowly, and the patients are monitored carefully during its administration.

Pulmonary Care

This aspect of therapy is often somewhat slighted. Change in position of these patients is frequently difficult because of the severity of the patient's illness and, in addition, because of the respirator, the various catheters, tubes and monitoring devices which are attached. On the other hand, a study from Dr. Spencer and his group has demonstrated that significant improvements in oxygenation can be obtained by frequent changes in position.[17] The corollary is that absence of change of position is likely to compound pulmonary problems, and this is supported by a variety of experimental work.[99]

In addition, routine pulmonary toilet, suctioning with sterile technique and attempts to prevent pulmonary infection are extremely important, but are sometimes neglected in the face of all the concomitant therapy which must be rendered to these patients. Such oversights can be lessened by establishing a flow sheet for turning, suctioning, and so on, with a check list for the nursing personnel to mark when these various measures are accomplished.

Drugs

In addition to the various medications which are used with ventilatory therapy, such as sedatives, narcotics and muscle relaxants, several drugs have been proposed as specifically efficacious for the treatment of pulmonary insufficiency. These include diuretics, steroids and heparin.

1. Diuretics.   Several published studies report improvement in hypoxic patients with intravenous administration of diuretics, particularly furosemide and ethycrinic acid.[29, 30, 75, 89] Many of these studies do not separate patients with acute pulmonary edema from those with progressive post-traumatic pulmonary insufficiency. The reports which *do* make this distinction demonstrate short-term improvement in arterial oxygenation in patients with fairly clear-cut post-traumatic pulmonary insufficiency. Frequently the improvement of oxygenation precedes any clinical evidence of diuresis, and, although it is generally thought that improvement is secondary to the diuresis, it well may be that some as yet undefined effect on the pulmonary capillary membrane is responsible for this improvement. It has been our practice to use moderate amounts of furosemide intravenously for short periods of time, particularly in the patient who exhibits hypoxia accompanied by fluid overload or signs of congestive heart failure. Many of these patients respond briskly and do not undergo progressive post-traumatic pulmonary insufficiency.

The use of long-term diuretic therapy with its attendant urine sodium loss, electrolyte imbalance and potential volume depletion is discouraged. Again, diuretics are not used in attempts to "dry out" the patients.

2. Steroids.   Dr. James Wilson and others have proposed the use of high doses of steroids as specific therapy in post-traumatic pulmonary insufficiency.[102] These recommendations are largely based on animal studies, but, as previously stated, most animal studies suffer from the lack of an appropriate model. The changes in animal studies upon which these recommendations are based are largely anatomical, and demonstrations of functional improvement in animal models with steroid therapy are sparse. Most of the studies which do show improvement use intravenous injection of fat or acid aspiration as a model. Patient data supporting the clinical use of steroids for post-traumatic pulmonary insufficiency are not yet available.

It is our feeling that the general application of high-dose steroids in these patients is not yet established as an appropriate therapeutic measure and carries with it complications which outweigh any presently supported benefits. On the other hand, we do institute short-term steroid therapy in patients immediately after aspiration of gastric juice, in the therapy of fat embolic syndrome and in patients with septic shock.

3. Heparin.   Suggestive evidence has been presented that heparin in appropriate doses benefits patients who suffer post-traumatic pulmonary insufficiency secondary to massive microembolism or intravascular coagulation.[13, 72] When one of these causative factors can be definitely incriminated, the use of moderate doses of heparin seems justified. High doses of heparin in patients with multiple injuries carry a significant potential risk. The ideal dose under these circumstances remains to be established.[72] We presently give doses in the range of 5,000 to 10,000 units every six hours.

The use of anticoagulation is restricted to the situations described above, since the beneficial effects of its application to all patients with post-traumatic pulmonary insufficiency have not been shown to outweigh its risk.

4. Antibiotics. Most of these patients are on antibiotics for various reasons, but their beneficial effect on the syndrome itself is yet to be established, and if other indications are not present, antibiotics are not given.

Summary

In summary, the syndrome of post-traumatic pulmonary insufficiency seems to be one of multiple causes, many of which are definable. The main thrust of therapy is ventilatory support until the patient recovers from his primary insult. In such a situation an aggressive attempt to define the cause of the pulmonary insufficiency is carried out while supportive therapy is going on. Therapy directed at resolving the specific cause is instituted when such can be identified. In our experience and in that of others, sepsis from either recognized or unrecognized causes appears to be the most common problem.

The ultimate form of supportive therapy, an extracorporeal pump oxygenator, is still in an embryonic stage. Significant work on a variety of pump oxygenators suitable for long-term support is under way.[40, 54] At present these are available only in a few centers and must, of necessity, be considered experimental.

REFERENCES

1. Ashbaugh, D. G., Bigelow, D. B., Petty, T. L., and Levine, B. E.: Acute respiratory distress in adults. Lancet, 2:7511, 1967.
2. Bates, D. V., Macklem, P. T., and Christie, R. V. (Editors): The Normal Lung: Physiology and Methods of Study. In Respiratory Function in Disease. Philadelphia, W. B. Saunders Company, 1971, Chap. 2.
3. Baue, A. E.: The Pushmi-pullyu syndrome. Surgery, 72:655, 1972.
4. Berman, I. R., and Ducker, T. B.: Pulmonary, somatic and splanchnic circulatory responses to increased intracranial pressure. Ann. Surg., 169:210, 1969.
5. Blaisdell, F. W., Lim, R. C., Jr., and Stallone, R. J.: The mechanism of pulmonary damage following traumatic shock. Surg., Gynec. Obstet., 130:15, 1970.
6. Boyd, D. R.: Monitoring patients with post-traumatic pulmonary insufficiency. Surg. Clin. N. Amer., 52:31, 1972.
7. Bredenberg, C. E., et al.: Respiratory failure in shock. Ann. Surg., 169:392, 1969.
8. Buckberg, G. D., and Dowell, A. R.: The effects of hemorrhagic shock and pulmonary ischemia on lung compliance and structure in baboons. Surg., Gynec. Obstet., 131:1065, 1970.

9. Buckberg, G. D., Lipman, C. A., Hahn, J. A., Smith, M. J., and Hennessen, J. A.: Pulmonary changes following hemorrhagic shock and resuscitation in baboons. J. Thorac. Cardiovasc. Surg., 59:450, 1970.

10. Burford, T. H., and Burbank, B.: Traumatic wet lung. Observations on certain physiologic fundamentals of thoracic trauma. J. Thorac. Surg., 14:415, 1945.

11. Burke, J. F., Pontoppidan, H., and Welch, C. E.: High output respiratory failure: An important cause of death ascribed to peritonitis or ileus. Ann. Surg., 158:581, 1963.

12. Burnham, S. C., Martin, W. E., and Cheney, F. W., Jr.: The effects of various tidal volumes on gas exchange in pulmonary edema. Anesthesiology, 37:27, 1972.

13. Cafferata, H. T., Aggeler, P. M., Robinson, A. J., and Blaisdell, F. W.: Intravascular coagulation in the surgical patient. Amer. J. Surg., 118:281, 1969.

14. Camerson, J. L., Anderson, R. P., and Zuidema, G. D.: Aspiration and pneumonia. A clinical and experimental review. J. Surg. Res., 7:44, 1967.

15. Carey, L. C., Lowery, B. D., and Cloutier, C. T.: Hemorrhagic Shock. Curr. Probl. Surg., Monograph, Jan., 1971.

16. Churchill, E. D.: Pulmonary atelectasis: With especial reference to massive collapse of lung. Arch. Surg., 11:489, 1925.

17. Clauss, R. H., Scalabrini, B. Y., Ray, J. F., II, and Reed, G. E.: Effects of Changing Body Position upon Improved Ventilation-Perfusion Relationships. Suppl. II to Circulation, 37 & 38:II-214, 1968.

18. Clowes, G. H. A., Jr., Farrington, G. H., Zuschneid, W., Cossette, G. R., and Saravis, C.: Circulating factors in the etiology of pulmonary insufficiency and right heart failure accompanying severe sepsis (peritonitis). Ann. Surg., 171:663, 1970.

19. Clowes, G. H. A., Jr., et al.: Observations on the pathogenesis of the pneumonitis associated with severe infections in other parts of the body. Ann. Surg., 167:630, 1968.

20. Coalson, J. J., Hinshaw, L. B., and Guenter, C. A.: The pulmonary ultrastructure in septic shock. Exp. Molec. Path., 12:84, 1970.

21. Collings, J. A.: The causes of progressive pulmonary insufficiency in surgical patients. J. Surg. Res., 9:685, 1969.

22. Collins, J. A., et al.: Inapparent hypoxemia in casualties with wounded limbs: Pulmonary fat embolism? Ann. Surg., 167:511, 1968.

23. Comroe, J. H., Jr., Forster, R. E., II, Dubois, A. B., Briscoe, W. A., and Carlsen, E. (Editors): The Pulmonary Circulation and Ventilation/Blood Flow Ratios. In The Lung, Clinical Physiology and Pulmonary Function Tests. Chicago, Year Book Medical Publishers, 1962, Chap. 4.

24. Ducker, T. B.: Increased intracranial pressure and pulmonary edema. Part I: Clinical study of 11 patients. J. Neurosurg., 28:112, 1968.

25. Eaton, R. M.: Pulmonary edema. Experimental observation on dogs following acute peripheral blood loss. J. Thorac. Surg., 16:668, 1947.

26. Eiseman, B., and Ashbaugh, D. G. (Editors): Pulmonary Effects of Nonthoracic Trauma. Proceedings of a Conf. Conducted by The Committee on Trauma, Div. of Med. Sciences, National Academy of Sciences – National Research Council. J. Trauma, Vol. 8, 1968.

27. Elliott, T. R., and Dingley, L. A.: Massive collapse of the lungs following abdominal operation. Lancet, 1:1305, 1914.

28. Falke, K. J., et al.: Ventilation with end-expiratory pressure in acute lung disease. J. Clin. Invest., 51:2315, 1972.

29. Fleming, W. H., and Bowen, J. C.: The use of diuretics in the treatment of early wet lung syndrome. Ann. Surg., 175:505, 1972.

30. Geiger, J. P., and Gielchinsky, I.: Acute pulmonary insufficiency. Arch. Surg., 102:400, 1971.

31. Gerst, P. H., Rattenborg, C., and Holday, D. A.: The effects of hemorrhage on pulmonary circulation and respiratory gas exchange. J. Clin. Invest., 38:524, 1959.

32. Gotoh, F., Meyer, J., and Takagi, Y.: Cerebral effects of hyperventilation in man. Arch. Neurol., 12:419, 1965.

33. Greenfield, L. J.: Pulmonary Dysfunction in Shock. In L. B. Hinshaw and B. G.

Cox (Editors): The Fundamental Mechanisms of Shock: Advances in Experimental Medicine and Biology. New York, Publ. Plenum Press, 1972, Vol. 23, p. 47.

34. Guenter, C. A., Fiorica, V., and Hinshaw, L. B.: Cardiorespiratory and metabolic responses to live *E. coli* and endotoxin in the monkey. J. Appl. Physiol., 26:780, 1969.

35. Gump, F. E., Mashima, Y., Ferenczy, A., and Kinney, J. M.: Pre- and postmortem studies of lung fluids and electrolytes. J. Trauma, 11:474, 1971.

36. Halmagyi, D. F. J., Goodman, A. H., Little, M. J., Kennedy, M., and Varga, D.: Portal blood flow and oxygen usage in dogs after hemorrhage. Ann. Surg., 172:284, 1970.

37. Hedden, M., and Miller, G. J.: Mendelson's syndrome and its sequelae. Canad. Anaesth. Soc. J., 19:351, 1972.

38. Henry, J. N., McArdle, A. H., Scott, H. J., and Gurd, F. N.: A study of the acute and chronic respiratory pathophysiology of hemorrhagic shock. J. Thorac. Cardiovasc. Surg., 54:666, 1967.

39. Herndon, J. H., Riseborough, E. J., and Fischer, J. E.: Fat embolism: A review of current concepts. J. Trauma, 11:673, 1971.

40. Hill, J. D., et al.: Acute respiratory insufficiency. Treatment with prolonged extracorporeal oxygenation. J. Thorac. Cardiovasc. Surg., 64:551, 1972.

41. Hillen, G. P., Gaisford, W. D., and Jensen, C. G.: Pulmonary changes in treated and untreated hemorrhagic shock. I. Early functional and ultrastructural alterations after moderate shock. Amer. J. Surg., 122:639, 1971.

42. Hinshaw, L. B., Emerson, T. E., Jr., and Reins, D. A.: Cardiovascular responses of the primate in endotoxin shock. Amer. J. Physiol., 210:335, 1966.

43. Hirsch, E. F., Fletcher, R., and Lucas, S.: Hemodynamic and respiratory changes associated with sepsis following combat trauma. Ann. Surg., 174:211, 1971.

44. Horovitz, J. H., and Carrico, C. J.: Lung colloid permeability in hemorrhagic shock. Surg. Forum, 23:6, 1972.

45. Horovitz, J. H., Carrico, C. J., Maher, J., and Shires, G. T.: Pulmonary shunt determination: A comparison between oxygen inhalation (Berggren) and xenon-133 methods. J. Lab. Clin. Med., 78:785, 1971.

46. Horovitz, J. H., Carrico, C. J., and Shires, G. T.: The pulmonary response to major injury. Submitted to Arch. of Surgery.

47. Huller, T., and Bazini, Y.: Blast injuries of the chest and abdomen. Arch. Surg., 100:24, 1970.

48. Jenkins, M. T., Jones, R. F., Wilson, B., and Moyer, C. A.: Congestive atelectasis — A complication of the intravenous infusion of fluids. Ann. Surg., 132:327, 1950.

49. Kafer, E. R.: Pulmonary oxygen toxicity. A review of the evidence for acute and chronic oxygen toxicity in man. Brit. J. Anaesth., 43:687, 1971.

50. Keller, C. A., Schramel, R. J., Hyman, A. L., and Creech, O., Jr.: The cause of acute congestive lesions of the lung. J. Thorac. Cardiovasc. Surg., 53:743, 1967.

51. Kim, S. I., Desai, J. M., and Shoemaker, W. C.: Sequential respiratory changes in an experimental hemorrhagic shock preparation designed to simulate clinical shock. Ann. Surg., 170:166, 1969.

52. Kumar, A., et al.: Continuous positive-pressure ventilation in acute respiratory failure. Effects on hemodynamics and lung function. New Eng. J. Med., 283:1430, 1970.

53. Laennec, R. T. H.: De l'auscultation médiate ou traité du diagnostic des maladies des poumons et du coeur, fondé principalement sur ce nouveau moyen d'exploration. Paris, 1819.

54. Lande, A. J., et al.: Prolonged cardio-pulmonary support with a practical membrane oxygenator. Trans. Amer. Soc. Artif. Intern. Organs, 16:352, 1970.

55. Levine, M., Gilbert, R., and Auchingloss, J. H., Jr.: A comparison of the effects of signs, large tidal volumes, and positive end expiratory pressure in assisted ventilation. Scand. J. Resp. Dis., 53:101, 1972.

56. Lim, R. C., Jr., Blaisdell, F. W., Choy, S. H., Goodman, J. R., and Hall, A. D.: Pulmonary microvascular changes following regional shock. A clinical and experimental study. Bull. Soc. Int. Chir., 1:22, 1968.

57. Markello, R., Winter, P., and Olszowka, A.: Assessment of ventilation-perfusion

inequalities by arterial-alveolar nitrogen differences in intensive-care patients. Anesthesiology, 37:4, 1972.

58. Martin, A. M., Jr., Soloway, H. B., and Simmons, R. L.: Pathologic anatomy of the lungs following shock and trauma. J. Trauma, 8:687, 1968.

59. McLaughlin, J. S.: Physiologic consideration of hypoxemia in shock and trauma. Ann. Surg., 173:667, 1971.

60. McNamara, J. J., Molot, M. D., and Stremple, J. F.: Screen filtration pressure in combat casualties. Ann. Surg., 172:334, 1970.

61. Michenfelder, J., Fowler, W., and Theye, R.: CO_2 levels and pulmonary shunting in anesthetized man. J. Appl. Physiol., 21:1471, 1966.

62. Mills, M.: The clinical syndrome. J. Trauma, 8:651, 1968.

63. Monaco, V., et al.: Pulmonary venous admixture in injured patients. J. Trauma, 12:15, 1972.

64. Moore, F. D., et al.: Post-Traumatic Pulmonary Insufficiency. Philadelphia, W. B. Saunders Company, 1969.

65. Moseley, R. V., and Doty, D. B.: Changes in the filtration characteristics of stored blood. Ann. Surg., 171:329, 1970.

66. Moss, G., Staunton, C., and Stein, A. A.: Cerebral etiology of the "shock lung syndrome." J. Trauma, 12:885, 1972.

67. Motsay, G. J., Alho, A. V., Schultz, L. S., Dietzman, R. H., and Lillehei, R. C.: Pulmonary capillary permeability in the post-traumatic pulmonary insufficiency syndrome: Comparison of isogravimetric capillary pressures. Ann. Surg., 173:244, 1971.

68. Naimark, A., Dugard, A., and Rangno, R. E.: Regional pulmonary blood flow and gas exchange in hemorrhagic shock. J. Appl. Physiol., 25:301, 1968.

69. Nash, G., Bowen, J. A., and Langlinais, P. C.: "Respirator lung": A misnomer. Arch. Path., 21:234, 1971.

70. Neeley, W. A., et al.: Postoperative respiratory insufficiency: Physiological studies with therapeutic implications. Ann. Surg., 171:679, 1970.

71. Nichols, R. T., Pearce, H. J., and Greenfield, L. J.: Effects of experimental pulmonary contusion on respiratory exchange and lung mechanics. Arch. Surg., 96:723, 1968.

72. Olcott, C., Barber, R. E., and Blaisdell, F. W.: Diagnosis and treatment of respiratory failure after civilian trauma. Amer. J. Surg., 122:260, 1971.

73. Pierce, A. K., Sanford, J. P., Thomas, G. D., and Leonard, J. S.: Long-term evaluation of decontamination of inhalation-therapy equipment and the occurrence of necrotizing pneumonia. New Eng. J. Med., 282:528, 1970.

74. Pinardi, G., Leal, E., and Sallas Coll, A.: Vascular permeability to red blood cells and protein in hemorrhagic shock. Acta. Physiol. Lat. Amer., 17:175, 1967.

75. Pontoppidan, H., Geffin, B., and Lowenstein, E.: Acute respiratory failure in the adult. New Eng. J. Med., 287:690, 1972.

76. Pontoppidan, H., Laver, M. B., and Geffin, B.: Acute respiratory failure in the surgical patient. Advances Surg., 4:163, 1970.

77. Powers, S. R., Jr., et al.: Studies of pulmonary insufficiency in non-thoracic trauma. J. Trauma, 12:1, 1972.

78. Proctor, H. J., Ballantine, T. V. N., and Broussard, N. D.: An analysis of pulmonary function following non-thoracic trauma, with recommendations for therapy. Ann. Surg., 172:180, 1970.

79. Robin, E. D., Carey, L. C., Grenvik, A., Glauser, F., and Gaudio, R.: Capillary leak syndrome with pulmonary edema. Arch. Intern. Med., 130:66, 1972.

80. Rounthwaite, H. L., Scott, H. J., and Gurd, F. N.: Changes in the pulmonary circulation during hemorrhagic shock and resuscitation. Surg. Forum, 3:454, 1952.

81. Said, S. I., et al.: Pulmonary gas exchange during induction of pulmonary edema in anesthetized dogs. J. Appl. Physiol., 19:403, 1964.

82. Schloerb, P. R., Hunt, P. T., Plummer, J. A., and Cage, G. K.: Pulmonary edema after replacement of blood loss by electrolyte solutions. Surg., Gynec., Obstet., 135:893, 1972.

83. Schon, G. R., Delpin, E. S., Millan, P. R., and Labat, R.: Relationship of blood substitutes to pulmonary changes and volemia. Ann. Surg., 173:504, 1971.

84. Sealy, W. C., Ogino, S., Lesage, A. M., and Young, W. G., Jr.: Functional and structural changes in the lungs in hemorrhagic shock. Surg., Gynec., Obstet., 122:754, 1966.
85. Siegel, D. C., Cochin, A., and Moss, G. S.: The ventilatory response to hemorrhagic shock and resuscitation. Surgery, 72:451, 1972.
86. Siegel, D. C., Moss, G. S., Cochin, A., and Das Gupta, T. K.: Pulmonary changes following treatment for hemorrhagic shock: Saline versus colloid infusion. Surg. Forum, 21:17, 1970.
87. Simeone, F. A.: Shock. In Christopher's Textbook of Surgery. Philadelphia, W. B. Saunders Company, 1964, p. 58.
88. Simmons, R. L., Martin, A. M., Jr., Heisterkamp, C. A., III, and Ducker, T. B.: Respiratory insufficiency in combat casualties: II. Pulmonary edema following head injury. Ann. Surg., 170:39, 1969.
89. Skillman, J. J., Parikh, B. M., and Tanenbaum, B. J.: Pulmonary arteriovenous admixture improvement with albumin and diuresis. Amer. J. Surg., 119:450, 1970.
90. Sladen, A., Laver, M. B., and Pontoppidan, H.: Pulmonary complications and water retention in prolonged mechanical ventilation. New Eng. J. Med., 279:448, 1968.
91. Stallone, R. J., Herbst, H., Blaisdell, F. W., and Murray, J. F.: Pulmonary changes following ischemia of the lower extremities and their treatment. Amer. Rev. Resp. Dis., 100:813, 1969.
92. Sterling, G. M.: The mechanism of bronchoconstriction due to hypocapnia in man. Clin. Sci., 34:277, 1968.
93. Sugg, W. F., et al.: Congestive atelectasis: An experimental study. Ann. Surg., 168:234, 1968.
94. Swank, R. L.: Alteration of blood on storage: Measurement of adhesiveness of "aging" platelets and leukocytes and their removal by filtration. New Eng. J. Med., 265:728, 1961.
95. Sykes, M. P., Adams, A. P., Finlay, W. E. I., Wightman, A. E., and Munroe, J. P.: The cardiorespiratory effects of haemorrhage and overtransfusion in dogs. Brit. J. Anaesth., 42:573, 1970.
96. Terzi, R. G., and Peters, R. M.: The effect of large fluid loads on lung mechanics and work. Ann. Thorac. Surg., 6:16, 1968.
97. Trimble, C., Smith, D. E., Rosenthal, M. H., and Fosburg, R. G.: Pathophysiologic role of hypocarbia in post-traumatic pulmonary insufficiency. Amer. J. Surg., 122:633, 1971.
98. Wahrenbrock, E. A., Carrico, C. J., Amundsen, D. A., Trummer, M. J., and Severinghaus, J. W.: Increased atelectatic pulmonary shunt during hemorrhagic shock in dogs. J. Appl. Physiol., 29:615, 1970.
99. Wahrenbrock, E. A., Carrico, C. J., Schroeder, C. F., and Trummer, M. J.: The effect of posture on pulmonary function and survival of anesthetized dogs. J. Surg. Res., 10:13, 1970.
100. Wangensteen, O. D., Wittmers, L. E., and Johnson, J. A.: Permeability of the mammalian blood-gas barrier and its components. Amer. J. Physiol., 216:719, 1969.
101. Willwerth, B. M., Crawford, F. A., Young, W. G., Jr., and Sealy, W. C.: The role of functional demand on the development of pulmonary lesions during hemorrhagic shock. J. Thorac. Cardiovasc. Surg., 54:658, 1967.
102. Wilson, J. W.: Treatment or prevention of pulmonary cellular damage with pharmacologic doses of corticosteroid. Surg., Gynec., Obstet., 134:675, 1972.
103. Wilson, R. F., Kafi, A., Asuncion, Z., and Walt, A. J.: Clinical respiratory failure after shock or trauma. Arch. Surg., 98:539, 1969.
104. Wyche, M. Q., Marshall, B. E., Mehall, S. L., and Schuetze, M. M.: Lung function, pulmonary extravascular water volume and hemodynamics in early hemorrhagic shock in anesthetized dogs. Ann. Surg., 174:296, 1971.

Chapter Five

ALTERATIONS IN
OXYGEN TRANSPORT

Cell hypoxia and eventually cell death may result from the complex changes induced by shock, regardless of the type, and efforts to restore delivery of oxygen to the tissues at an adequate concentration and pressure form the basis for treatment. In the past, attention was directed primarily toward the factors affecting oxygen transport capability, including the concentration and partial pressure of oxygen in the inspired air, alveolar ventilation, ventilation-perfusion relationships, cardiac output, blood volume and hemoglobin concentration. The recent demonstration that the level of organic phosphates in the red blood cell has a significant effect on the position of the oxygen-hemoglobin dissociation curve has served to focus attention on the processes responsible for release of oxygen at the tissue level. Because of the clinical implication of these findings, a knowledge of factors regulating both oxygen uptake and release has assumed increasing importance in the care of critically ill patients.

OXYGEN TRANSPORT

The oxygen transport system consists of several component processes that function collectively to extract oxygen from inspired air and deliver it at a partial pressure sufficient to allow rapid diffusion from blood into the body cells. Each of the component processes has its own internal controls, and failure of any one may be compensated by

97

adjustments in the remainder of the system. The functions of the oxygen transport system are summarized in the following formula:

Oxygen consumption =

$$\text{Arteriovenous oxygen content difference} \times \frac{\text{Cardiac output (L/min.)}}{100}$$

The amount of oxygen in whole blood includes that bound to hemoglobin (1.38 ml O_2/gm of hemoglobin) and a small amount dissolved in plasma (0.003 ml/mm of oxygen tension). The oxygen content of arterial (Ca_{O_2}) and venous blood ($C\bar{v}_{O_2}$) are calculated by the formula:

$$\text{Oxygen content} = 1.38 \times \text{Hgb. conc.} \times \text{Hgb. sat.} + 0.003 \times P_{O_2}$$

Consider a person with a hemoglobin of 15 gm per 100 ml, an arterial oxygen tension of 100 mm Hg, a venous oxygen tension of 40 mm Hg, arterial and venous hemoglobin saturations of 97 and 75 per cent respectively, and a cardiac output of 6 L/min. Substituting these values in the formulas above, arterial oxygen content is 20.4 vols. per 100 ml, venous oxygen content is 15.6 vols. per 100 ml, arteriovenous oxygen difference is 4.8 vols. per 100 ml, and oxygen consumption is 288 ml/min.

Changes in any one of these factors are of variable significance regarding oxygen delivery. For instance, pulmonary gas exchange with 20 per cent inspired oxygen concentration ($F_{I_{O_2}}$) normally produces an arterial oxygen tension (Pa_{O_2}) of approximately 100 mm Hg, slightly less than average alveolar oxygen tension. Increasing the $F_{I_{O_2}}$ to 100 per cent would raise Pa_{O_2} to approximately 650 mm Hg. This would increase the amount of dissolved oxygen in the plasma from 0.3 to 2.0 vols. per 100 ml, but would only increase the hemoglobin saturation from 97 to 100 per cent. In contrast, even moderate changes in hemoglobin concentration or cardiac output have a strong influence on oxygen transport capability. A hemoglobin concentration of 10 gm per 100 ml (instead of 15) in the patient example above would reduce oxygen-carrying capacity of the blood by one third (Ca_{O_2} — 13.7 vols. per 100 ml). Coupled with a fall in cardiac output from 6 to 3 L/min., assuming that other variables remain unchanged, oxygen consumption theoretically would fall from 288 to 96 ml/min. This is not an infrequent clinical occurrence, although oxygen consumption would be maintained at a higher level by adjustments in other parts of the system (e.g. increase of arteriovenous oxygen difference).

Therapy designed to improve tissue oxygenation, therefore, includes an evaluation of all factors affecting the oxygen transport system. Adjustment of inspired oxygen concentration and efforts to improve alveolar ventilation are of obvious importance; however, therapeutic attempts to maintain a normal hemoglobin concentration and cardiac output deserve special attention.[33]

OXYGEN-HEMOGLOBIN DISSOCIATION CURVE

Another aspect of oxygen transport which deserves emphasis is the relationship between hemoglobin oxygen saturation and oxygen tension. The oxyhemoglobin dissociation curve describes hemoglobin affinity for oxygen, and its unusual sigmoid shape reflects the phenomenon of heme-heme interaction. Each of four heme groups in the hemoglobin molecule reacts with oxygen in a prescribed order, and uptake of an oxygen molecule by one heme group facilitates the oxygenation of the next heme group. The sigmoid configuration of this curve is particularly suitable for the uptake, transport and subsequent release of oxygen. Since the upper portion of the dissociation curve is relatively flat, oxygen loading by hemoglobin may remain relatively normal despite wide variations in the alveolar oxygen tension. As oxygenated blood traverses the peripheral capillary, however, PO_2 drops from approximately 100 to 40 mm Hg, hemoglobin saturation falls from 97 to 75 per cent, and the blood releases just over 22 per cent of its oxygen load (Fig. 5–1). Since PO_2 values at the peripheral capillary level fall on the steep portion of the curve, significant changes in oxygen release are produced by only small alterations in oxygen tension.

The position of the oxyhemoglobin dissociation curve along the horizontal axis is characteristically termed the P_{50} value (Fig. 5–1). This reflects the oxygen tension necessary to saturate 50 per cent of the hemoglobin with oxygen; the normal value is approximately 27 mm Hg.

The importance of positional changes of the curve is also related to its sigmoid shape. Within limits, rightward or leftward shifts have little effect on arterial oxygen saturation if Pa_{O_2} is above 80 mm Hg. At the peripheral capillary level, however, even small shifts of the curve may be important. A rightward shift of the dissociation curve (P_{50} above 27 mm Hg) indicates decreased hemoglobin affinity for oxygen, while a leftward shift (P_{50} below 27 mm Hg) is associated with an increase of hemoglobin-oxygen affinity. Compared to the normally positioned curve, more oxygen is released at any given PO_2 with a rightward-shifted curve and less is released with a leftward-shifted curve. Therefore, if arterial and venous oxygen tensions remain constant, arteriovenous oxygen difference increases with a rightward shift of the curve and decreases with a leftward shift (Fig. 5–2).

Changes in position of the oxygen-hemoglobin dissociation curve

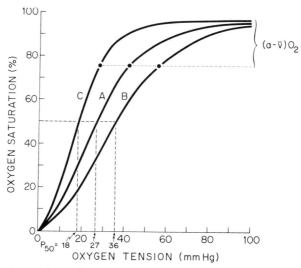

Figure 5–1 Oxygen-hemoglobin dissociation curves in *(A)* normal, *(B)* rightward shifted and *(C)* leftward-shifted positions. The P_{50} value denotes the position of the curve along the horizontal axis and represents the oxygen tension (in mm. Hg) necessary to saturate 50 per cent of available hemoglobin with oxygen. Note that as the curve moves toward the left, the arteriovenous oxygen difference, $(a-\bar{v})O_2$, can be maintained only by decreasing venous oxygen tension. (Adapted from S. D. Shappell and C. J. M. Lenfant: Adaptive, genetic, and iatrogenic alterations of the oxyhemoglobin-dissociation curve. Anesthesiology, 37:127, 1972.)

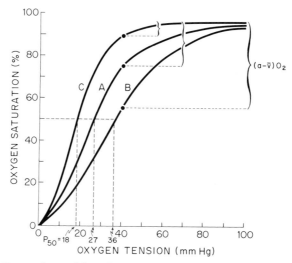

Figure 5–2 Oxygen-hemoglobin dissociation curves similar to those in Figure 5–1. Note that if arterial and venous oxygen tensions remain constant, arteriovenous oxygen difference decreases as the curve moves toward the left.

are significant in at least two respects. The transfer of oxygen from the blood to the sites of intracellular utilization is directly related to the oxygen pressure differential. Thus a rightward shift of the curve is theoretically advantageous, since an equivalent amount of oxygen is released at a higher PO_2 than with a leftward-positioned curve. (Note that in curve B of Figure 5–1, half of the oxygen would be released at a PO_2 of 36 mm Hg; in curve C less than 10 per cent of the oxygen would be released at the same PO_2.) Secondly, the ability to maintain or enlarge the arteriovenous oxygen difference is dependent to some extent on the position of the curve. Normally, arterial hemoglobin saturation is near the upper limit and cannot be increased appreciably. Any enlargement of the arteriovenous oxygen difference necessitates reduction in venous hemoglobin saturation and venous oxygen tension $P\overline{v}_{O_2}$). As the curve moves to the left, maintenance of any given arteriovenous oxygen difference requires a progressive decrease in $P\overline{v}_{O_2}$. The fall in $P\overline{v}_{O_2}$ is finally limited by the fact that a certain partial pressure is necessary for transfer of oxygen from the blood to the tissue cell. That level of oxygen pressure below which diffusion may be theoretically impaired and cellular function disturbed has been termed the "critical PO_2."[24]

Available data concerning the critical PO_2 are limited, but suggest that it varies in individual organ systems and may depend on the level of activity of the tissues. Opitz and Snyder showed that oxygen uptake by the brain is impaired when venous oxygen tension falls below 20 to 25 mm Hg,[23] while Berne et al. indicated loss of myocardial function at oxygen tensions between 10 and 12 mm Hg.[4] With a leftward movement of the curve, therefore, maintaining or enlarging the arteriovenous oxygen difference is theoretically limited as the $P\overline{v}_{O_2}$ approaches this critical level. Tissue oxygen delivery may be sustained in this instance by other mechanisms, principally by increasing cardiac output.

During hypovolemic shock, cardiac output is low and relatively fixed. Normally, enlargement of arteriovenous oxygen difference will partially compensate for the diminished blood flow; however, the response may be totally inadequate with a leftward shift of the dissociation curve. Continued survival and maintenance of essential organ function may be obtained only by shunting blood from tissues that tolerate a limited period of severe hypoxia (skin, skeletal muscle) to organs that require high oxygen flow rates (brain, heart).

Factors Influencing the Position of the Oxygen-Hemoglobin Dissociation Curve

Attempts to ensure a normal or rightward-positioned dissociation curve may be essential during treatment of patients with low-flow states. Factors affecting the position of the curve have been summarized recently by Shappel and Lenfant and are outlined in Table 5–1.[31] The main in-vivo influences include changes in pH, temperature, partial pressure of carbon dioxide and the level of red blood cell organic phosphates. Changes in hydrogen ion concentration and temperature have predictable and instantaneous effects on the position of the curve, while P_{CO_2} exerts its influence both by changing pH and by a pH-independent effect.[22, 28] The quantitative effects of these influences on the dissociation curve have been reviewed in several excellent publications.[2, 6, 29, 31]

Recent investigations by Chanutin and Curnish and by Benesch and Benesch indicate that the position of the dissociation curve is also influenced by interaction of hemoglobin with organic phosphates in the red blood cell.[3, 9] Both ATP and 2,3-diphosphoglycerate (DPG) bind to hemoglobin and lower the affinity of hemoglobin for oxygen, i.e. shift the dissociation curve to the right. In a quantitative sense, DPG is the more important of the two phosphates and exerts an additional influence in the intact red blood cell by lowering intracellular pH via Donnan equilibrium.[13] Significant concentrations of DPG are found only in the red blood cell, and DPG is present in approximately equimolar concentration to that of hemoglobin. DPG is a product of erythrocyte glycolysis, formed via a branch of the Embden-Myerhof pathway by conversion of 1,3-DPG to 2,3-DPG, catalyzed by diphosphoglycerate mutase (Fig. 5–3).

Erythrocyte DPG undergoes considerable changes in response

Table 5–1   Factors That Alter Hemoglobin — Oxygen Affinity

INCREASE P_{50}	DECREASE P_{50}
By direct effect	*By direct effect:*
Increased [H⁺]	Decreased [H⁺]
Temperature	Temperature
P_{CO_2}	P_{CO_2}
DPG, ATP	DPG, ATP
Hgb. conc.	Hgb. conc.
Ionic strength	Ionic strength
Abnormal hemoglobin	Abnormal hemoglobin
Aldosterone	Carboxyhemoglobin
	Methemoglobin
By increasing DPG:	*By decreasing DPG:*
Decreased [H⁺]	Increased [H⁺]
Thyroid hormone	Decreased thyroid hormone
Pyruvate kinase deficiency	Hexokinase deficiency
Increased inorganic phosphate	Decreased inorganic phosphate
Cortisol	Cell age (old)
Cell age (young)	

Adapted from S. D. Shappell, and C. J. M. Lenfant: Adaptive genetic and iatrogenic alterations of the oxyhemoglobin-dissociation curve. Anesthesiology, 37:127–139, 1971.

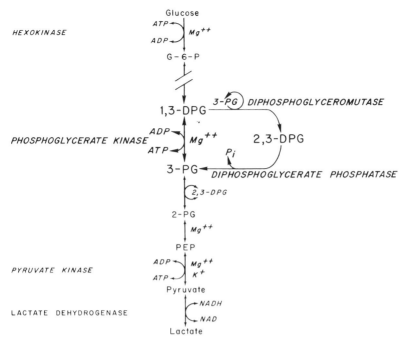

Figure 5–3   Glycolytic pathway of red blood cell. Note the formation of 2,3-diphospho-glycerate from 1,3-diphosphoglycerate, catalyzed by diphosphoglycerate mutase.

to several stimuli, with parallel changes in the position of the dissociation curve. Recent investigations have revealed that hypoxia increases erythrocyte DPG in conditions such as exercise, anemia, exposure to high altitude, cardiac failure and various pulmonary diseases.[17,18,20,21,34,36,40] The concomitant rightward shifts of the dissociation curve are thought to represent significant compensatory responses allowing release of more oxygen at a higher Po_2.

The regulation of DPG synthesis is complex and as yet not fully clarified. Although numerous factors influence the level of DPG (Table 5–1), the principal *mechanism* for increasing or decreasing its concentration appears to be related to the level of hydrogen ions in the red cell. DPG concentration increases as the red blood cell pH rises, and decreases as the pH falls. These changes are due, in part, to the differential effects of pH on the activity of two red cell enzymes, DPG mutase and phosphatase.[15] For instance, alkalosis stimulates DPG synthesis by increasing DPG-mutase activity and reducing the breakdown of DPG by DPG-phosphatase. The rise in red cell pH may be secondary to elevation of whole blood pH or, as in hypoxic states, a relative increase in the amount of deoxyhemoglobin.[2] PH also influences DPG binding to hemoglobin and may affect other enzymes in the glycolytic cycle.[6] The net effect of pH changes on DPG concentration, therefore, probably represents a combination of these (and other unknown) influences. It should be noted that the pH-induced changes in DPG concentration tend to counteract the direct pH effects on the curve via the Bohr effect. Therefore the immediate rightward shift of the curve secondary to acute acidosis is eventually offset by a pH-induced reduction in DPG concentration.

DPG synthesis is also responsive to hormonal influences and the level of inorganic phosphate. The phosphate level is directly related to DPG concentration, and maintenance of a normal inorganic phosphate level during intravenous hyperalimentation is necessary to prevent a reduction in the level of erythrocyte 2,3-DPG.[26] Thyroid hormone acts directly to increase DPG synthesis, a fact which probably explains the elevated levels of this compound in hyperthyroid patients.[32] Cortisol and aldosterone both shift the dissociation curve to the right, thereby decreasing hemoglobin-oxygen affinity.[1] The effects of cortisol are probably secondary to direct stimulation of DPG synthesis.[19] Hemoglobin-oxygen affinity also increases as the erythrocyte ages, presumably owing to a decreasing DPG concentration.[16]

BLOOD TRANSFUSIONS, ERYTHROCYTE DPG AND OXYGEN DELIVERY

The acceptability of blood (properly stored up to three weeks) for transfusion is based on the fact that at least 70 per cent of the transfused cells will survive in the recipient's circulation. During this period of time, however, hemoglobin-oxygen affinity of the stored cells slowly increases, and at the end of three weeks the oxygen dissociation curve is markedly shifted to the left. It is now well established that this phenomenon results from progressive depletion of DPG in blood stored in ACD solution.[5, 7, 10, 35] Depending on the quality of the transfused cells and the condition of the patient, it requires 24 hours or longer after transfusion before DPG levels return to normal.[8, 38] The possibility that oxygen transport may be seriously impaired in the massively transfused patient, particularly in the presence of inadequate or fixed low cardiac output, prompted several studies in the laboratory and Trauma Research Unit at Parkland Memorial Hospital.

Erythrocyte DPG levels were measured in 38 injured patients and seven patients with various surgical illnesses who received at least five units of whole blood during resuscitation and the operative procedure.[8] Attempts were made to correlate DPG concentration with

P_{50} (18 patients), mixed venous Po_2, arteriovenous oxygen difference and oxygen consumption.

Mean values for DPG concentration following initial transfusions, correlated with the amount and storage time of transfused whole blood, are shown in Table 5–2. The average storage time of blood given to these patients is high, and is consistent with the common economic practice employed by blood banks where the oldest compatible blood is issued first for use in transfusion. This is probably of little consequence with one or two unit transfusions, but may be significant after massive infusions of whole blood. In view of rapid depletion of this compound in stored blood, the depressed levels of DPG in these patients reflect a simple dilutional phenomenon. When the patient is actually bleeding during transfusion, however, the final level of DPG will depend primarily on the storage time of the last few units of blood infused. This point may assume clinical importance when dealing with an individual patient, as illustrated in Figure 5–4. During resuscitation from shock and the early part of the operative procedure the patient received 7,500 ml of whole blood with an average storage age of 12 days. The fall in DPG concentration which resulted was reversed near the end of the operative procedure by using fresh blood for the remainder of the required transfusions.

DPG levels were below normal in the majority of these patients; the lowest recorded value was 0.65 $\mu M/ml$ of red blood cells (normal range 4.5 to 5.0). There were no consistent correlations, however, between DPG concentration and the measured parameters of oxygen delivery. Oxygen consumption was reasonably well maintained in most of the patients, although in 12 instances (10 patients) the level fell below 65 ml/min./M^2. Corresponding DPG concentrations varied from 0.65 to 7.20 $\mu M/ml$ of red cells. Considering only those instances in which DPG concentrations were less than half normal, oxygen consumption varied between 40 and 340 ml/min./M^2. Four of the 10 patients with oxygen consumptions below 65 ml/min./M^2 died. Three of

Table 5–2   2,3-Diphosphoglycerate Concentration
Following Blood Transfusion

	2,3-DPG CONCENTRATION ($\mu M/ML.$ RBC)			
	<2	2.0–2.99	3.0–3.99	>3.99
Number of patients..........	12	9	19	5
Mean 2,3-DPG conc.........	1.14	2.57	3.42	4.26
Mean quantity of transfused blood (ml) ...	7,300	5,650	7,100	3,100
Mean storage age of blood (days).............	11.7	12.5	9.3	10.8

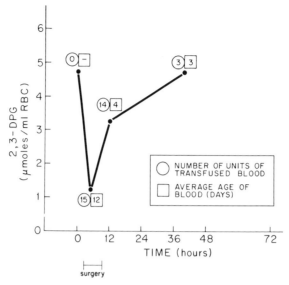

Figure 5–4 2,3-Diphosphoglycerate concentrations following whole blood transfusions in a patient with multiple bone fractures and a large stellate laceration of the liver requiring right hepatic lobectomy.

the four patients had normal or elevated DPG levels and normal or rightward-positioned dissociation curves.

The lack of correlation between DPG concentration and the measured parameters of oxygen delivery may be explained by two additional observations. First, the position of the dissociation curve cannot be reliably predicted from a knowledge of the DPG concentration alone (Fig. 5–5). DPG represents only one of several factors that affect the curve, and the final P_{50} represents a composite of these influences. Normal or elevated P_{50} values noted in several patients

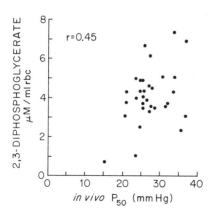

Figure 5–5 2,3-Diphosphoglycerate and in vivo P_{50} values in 18 patients (32 sets of determinations) after whole blood transfusions. Correlation coefficient, 0.45.

with low DPG concentrations were probably due to the presence of other factors (e.g. pH and temperature) which tended to counteract the influence of DPG. A second observation that may explain our inability to demonstrate a correlation between DPG concentration and oxygen delivery is the lack of a consistent relationship between the P_{50} value and oxygen consumption (Fig. 5–6). The majority of patients with left-ward shifts of the dissociation curve had reasonably normal arterio-venous oxygen differences and oxygen consumptions. Additionally, several of the patients with narrowed arteriovenous oxygen differ-ences maintained oxygen delivery simply by increasing the cardiac output.

These findings do not imply that the position of the dissociation curve and the factors that influence it was unimportant. They do sug-gest that a person with reasonably intact cardiovascular and pulmo-nary systems is able to tolerate rather significant leftward shifts of the oxygen dissociation curve. The consequences may be quite different, however, in a patient with limited compensatory mechanisms.

In an effort to clarify the relationship between oxygen consump-tion and the position of the oxygen dissociation curve, several studies are currently in progress. Because of the large number of variables present in the clinical situation, an experimental animal model has been developed. It consists of an exchange transfusion in a dog using compatible blood depleted of erythrocyte DPG. The result is a nor-motensive, normovolemic animal with an erythrocyte DPG concen-tration approximately 15 to 20 per cent of normal. Preliminary data from these studies indicate that a leftward shift of the dissociation curve may seriously hamper efforts to maintain oxygen delivery during hemorrhagic shock. Further, the use of some therapeutic regimens without a knowledge of their effects on the position of the curve may simply compound the problem. An example of this is illus-trated in Figure 5–7, in which the expected leftward shift of the

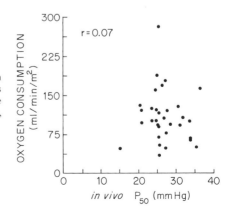

Figure 5–6 Oxygen consumption and in vivo P_{50} measurements in 18 patients (32 sets of determinations) after whole blood transfusions. Correlation coefficient, 0.07.

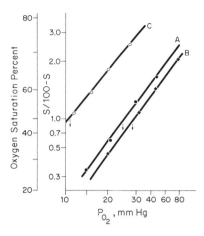

Figure 5–7 Oxygen-hemoglobin dissociation curves (plotted on log-log scales) in a dog during a control period (curve *A*, DPG 5.20 μM/ml RBC) and after exchange transfusion with DPG-depleted blood (curve *B*, DPG 0.74). The expected leftward shift secondary to low DPG concentration was effectively counteracted by the development of severe acidosis during the exchange transfusion. Note the decided leftward shift by the Bohr effect following alkalinization with sodium bicarbonate (curve *C*).

dissociation curve due to low erythrocyte DPG was effectively counteracted by the acidosis that developed during exchange transfusion. The sudden correction of pH to normal with sodium bicarbonate resulted in a decided leftward shift of the dissociation curve.

The potential importance of maintaining a normally positioned dissociation curve and hemoglobin concentration during hemorrhagic shock is shown in Figure 5–8. DPG concentration and the position of the dissociation curve were maintained in the control dog during an exchange transfusion with *fresh* blood, and oxygen consumption remained unaltered. The dog was then bled to a mean blood pressure of 50 mm Hg. Despite the sharp reduction in cardiac output, oxygen delivery was maintained at a reasonable level, since the arteriovenous oxygen difference increased from 4.5 to 10.6 ml. In contrast, the DPG-depleted dog was unable to expand the arteriovenous oxygen difference sufficiently (P_{50} value 15 mm Hg). The problem was compounded by attempts to correct pH to normal by infusion

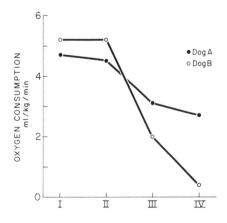

Figure 5–8 Effects of hemorrhagic shock and sodium bicarbonate infusion on oxygen consumption after exchange transfusion with fresh blood (dog A) and DPG-depleted blood (dog B). I, Control period; II, after exchange transfusion (DPG concentration 6.20 μM/ml RBC in dog A and 0.80 μM/ml RBC in dog B); III, after induction of hypotension; IV, continued hypotension and sodium bicarbonate infusion.

of sodium bicarbonate solution. The dissociation curve moved further to the left (P_{50} value 8 mm Hg), the hemoglobin concentration fell secondary to hemodilution, and oxygen consumption fell near zero. The level of excess lactate at this point was 16.5 mM/L (normal value 1 mM/L), and the dog expired shortly thereafter. The control dog survived, and at the conclusion of the experiment had an excess lactate level of 1.0. Although extreme, the experimental conditions are not unlike those that may be found in the clinical setting.

In summary, available evidence suggests that changes in hemoglobin-oxygen affinity, as reflected by the position of the oxygen dissociation curve, may be important in several circumstances. The elevated DPG concentrations and rightward shifts of the dissociation curve observed in hypoxic states (pulmonary disease, cardiac failure, anemia, exposure to high altitude, and so on) probably represent compensatory responses that facilitate oxygen unloading in the tissue capillaries. Maintenance of oxygenation in these instances can be accomplished by other mechanisms (e.g. increasing cardiac output), but at a greater expense to body economy.

Leftward shifts of the dissociation curve observed following transfusions of stored blood, acute alkalosis, hypothermia, and so forth, are, at best, undesirable phenomena and may significantly impair oxygen unloading. Although leftward shifts are tolerated in many circumstances, maintenance of a normally positioned dissociation curve may be of singular importance in patients with hypoxia, anemia or hypotension when compensatory responses are limited.

THERAPEUTIC IMPLICATIONS

The use of stored blood for massive blood replacement or exchange transfusion is increasing in frequency. The acceptability for transfusion of blood which has been stored in ACD solution for up to three weeks is based on survival of at least 70 per cent of the cells in the recipient's circulation. But during this three-week period there is a rapid decline in erythrocyte 2,3-diphosphoglycerate (DPG) and a progressive increase in hemoglobin-oxygen affinity (leftward shift of the oxygen dissociation curve).[5, 7, 10, 35] After transfusion it requires 24 hours or longer for the DPG levels to return to normal.[8, 38] These findings indicate that oxygen delivery may be impaired after the administration of large quantities of stored blood and have led to a re-evaluation of transfusion practices. Present knowledge suggests the use of limited quantities of older stored blood in patients with stabilized chronic diseases and the use of relatively fresh blood when possible in most acutely ill patients.[6]

An exchange transfusion in the newborn to reduce the bilirubin level is a well known indication for the use of fresh blood. Replacing fetal hemoglobin that has a left-shifted oxygen dissociation curve with fresh adult blood has also been advocated to enhance oxygen transport capability in premature infants with respiratory distress syndrome.[12] Similarly, the use of fresh blood is indicated when exchange transfusions are done for other purposes (e.g. hepatic coma), during elective surgery when a large blood loss is expected, and during cardiopulmonary bypass in cardiac surgery. This is particularly important in the last instance when hypothermia, acid-base changes and depressed myocardial function may sharply reduce oxygen delivery.

In most of these cases, there is sufficient time to obtain adequate quantities of fresh blood. For the treatment of hemorrhagic shock during emergency surgery or following injury, however, the physician must rely on available blood supplies, regardless of storage age. Obtaining an adequate quantity of blood is difficult in some areas, and even large blood banks have only limited supplies of fresh compatible blood. The solution to this problem will ultimately involve finding a satisfactory technique to preserve or rapidly restore the level of DPG in stored blood. Several methods have been proposed, including the addition of inosine and adenine to the storage media, storage of blood in a new artificial medium, and the use of frozen blood.[11, 37, 39] DPG is stable in the frozen state, and because of its other inherent advantages, freezing blood may be the ideal method for its preservation.

Successful in-vitro restoration of DPG concentration prior to transfusion has been reported recently by Oski et al.[25] and Duhm et al.[14] Both groups have been able to restore DPG and P_{50} levels to normal (and above) by incubating banked blood with inosine, inorganic phosphate and pyruvate. The use of methylprednisolone has also been reported to increase the concentration of DPG in stored blood.[19] Both methods require that blood be incubated several hours prior to transfusion. Other compounds, including methylene blue and sulfates, have been shown to affect the level of DPG in vivo, and Pollack et al. have recently reported increases of DPG concentration in experimental animals following the intravenous administration of inosine, inorganic phosphate and pyruvate.[27] Although one or more of these techniques may be useful in the near future, none have proved to be completely satisfactory.

At present, storage of blood in CPD (citrate-phosphate-dextrose) solution seems to be the most practical alternative. Survival of red blood cells is similar after transfusion of blood stored in either ACD or CPD solution. Compared to ACD solution, however, blood stored in CPD media has a higher pH, and DPG and P_{50} are maintained at consistently higher levels.[10, 30] Conversion from ACD to CPD solution for blood storage is a simple matter for blood banks, since CPD transfusion packs are currently available commercially at no increase in cost. The administration of limited quantities of older ACD- or CPD-stored blood in an acute situation is acceptable, although the full oxygen delivery capability of this blood may not be realized for several hours. When larger quantities of blood are administered, particularly in critically ill patients, the storage age of each unit should be recorded. If a significant portion of the blood administered is more than a few days old, every attempt should be made to obtain fresh blood for additional transfusion requirements. In our experience the institution of these simple changes has been rewarding. The large reductions in DPG and P_{50} noted in earlier studies are rarely seen today, even after massive transfusions.[8]

Consideration of other factors that influence the position of the dissociation curve (Table 5–1) may also be important in the individual patient. For instance, the induction of a respiratory alkalosis may produce an abrupt increase in hemoglobin-oxygen affinity. This is a common occurrence during operations and in patients requiring ventilatory assistance in the postoperative period; coupled with other factors that limit oxygen transport, the capacity to maintain tissue oxygenation may be sharply reduced. Similarly, the sudden correction of an acidosis, whether metabolic or respiratory, may have undesirable effects. In this regard the indiscriminate use of sodium bicarbonate during resuscitation of patients in hypovolemic shock is discouraged. The presence of a mild metabolic alkalosis is a common finding after resuscitation, owing in part to the alkalinizing effects of blood transfusions and the administration of lactated Ringer's solution. After infusion (and partial restoration of hepatic blood flow) the citrate and lactate contained in transfused blood and the lactate in lactated Ringer's solution are metabolized and bicarbonate is formed. If excessive quantities of sodium bicarbonate are administered simultaneously, a severe metabolic alkalosis may result. The alkaline pH may be highly undesirable, particularly in patients with hypoxia or low fixed cardiac output. Combined with other factors incident to blood replacement which increase hemoglobin-oxygen affinity (low DPG concentration and hypothermia), significant interference with oxygen unloading at the cellular level may occur.

The immediate and direct pH influences on the curve (via the Bohr effect) are eventually offset by reciprocal changes in DPG concentration. There is, however, a lag period of approximately four hours before any change in DPG concentration is noted, and the final level is not reached until 48 hours after induction of acidosis or alkalosis.[2] The fact that the effects of sudden large changes in pH may persist for several hours should be considered during therapy. Correction of a metabolic acidosis, therefore, is properly directed toward correction of the underlying disorder. Bicarbonate therapy may be reserved for the treatment of severe metabolic acidosis, particularly following cardiac arrest, when *partial* correction of pH is essential to restore myocardial function. Similarly, pH correction in more protracted states of metabolic acidosis may be indicated, but should be accomplished slowly.

Lowering body temperature also causes a leftward shift of the dissociation curve and an increase in hemoglobin-oxygen affinity, but any interference in oxygen delivery may be countered effectively by the hypothermia-induced reduction in metabolic requirements.

Rightward shifts of the curve are usually desirable and, unless extreme, rarely interfere with oxygen uptake in the lungs. Rightward shifts generally occur as a compensatory response to hypoxia, regardless of the cause. Nevertheless, in patients with severe arterial desaturation (exposure to high altitude, congestive failure, right-to-left cardiac shunts), any potential benefit from shifting the curve further to the right may be offset by interference with oxygen loading.[31]

In a complex clinical setting multiple factors that influence hemoglobin-oxygen affinity may be operative at any given time, and abrupt changes secondary to therapy or the disease process itself may occur. Evaluation of these multiple influences may be difficult, since few data concerning their cumulative effects are available. Nevertheless their *net* effect can be estimated by determining the position of the oxygen dissociation curve.

Techniques for constructing an oxygen dissociation curve are time-consuming and not readily available in most hospitals. For this reason we have developed a rapid, though less precise, method for estimating the position of the curve (the P_{50} value). Since the shape and slope of the curve do not change appreciably with changes in position, determination of a single point on the steep part of the slope should allow a rough estimate of the entire curve. To obviate the use of a tonometer, a single sample of venous blood is drawn anaerobically, and the PO_2 and oxygen saturation are measured (an arterial sample is unsuitable, since the values fall on the upper flat portion of the curve). An estimated P_{50} value may then be obtained using the Severinghaus slide rule* or a nomogram as depicted in Figure 5–9. The nomogram represents a computer plot of a family of O_2 dissociation curves using the correction factor for pH as suggested by Severinghaus.[29] The point on the nomogram corresponding to the measured PO_2 and saturation values is found and traced to the line representing 50 per cent oxygen saturation. This intersect represents the estimated P_{50}; the normal value is approximately 27 mm Hg. A

---

*Blood Gas Calculator, Type BGC-1 (Scales designed by J. W. Severinghaus, M. D.), Copyright 1967 by Radiometer A/S, Emdrupve 72, Copenhagen NV, Denmark.

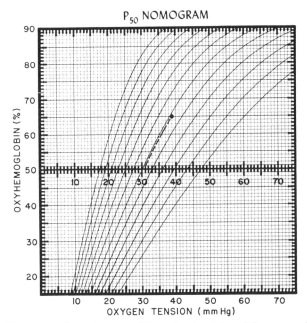

Figure 5–9 Nomogram for estimation of P_{50} value (position of the oxygen-hemoglobin dissociation curve). The point on the nomogram corresponding to the measured P_{O_2} and saturation of a sample of venous blood is traced to the line representing 50 per cent oxygen saturation. This intersect represents the estimated P_{50} (normal value approximately 27 mm Hg).

In the example shown, the venous blood sample P_{O_2} is 39 mm Hg, the oxygen saturation 65 per cent, and the P_{50} value is 31 mm Hg (a rightward positioned dissociation curve).

P_{50} above this level represents a rightward shift of the oxygen dissociation curve, while a lower value represents a leftward shift.

To test the validity of this technique, oxygen dissociation curves were constructed using a standard mixing technique on 50 occasions in 27 acutely ill patients. In each instance an estimated P_{50} was ob-

Figure 5–10 Comparison of the estimated P_{50} values (nomogram) with the determined P_{50} values (mixing chamber technique) in 27 acutely ill patients (50 sets of determinations; correlation coefficient 0.92).

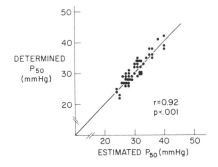

tained from the nomogram using a single sample of venous blood drawn at the same time. Correlation between the two values was excellent (correlation coefficient 0.92), as shown in Figure 5–10.

Estimates of P_{50} have become routine in our care of critically ill patients. Combined with measurements of both arterial and venous blood gases, a considerable amount of information may be obtained about the state of oxygenation and oxygen transport capability.

REFERENCES

1. Bauer, C. H., and Ratschlag-Schaefer, A. M.: The influence of aldosterone and cortisol on oxygen affinity and cation concentration of the blood. Resp. Physiol., 5:360, 1968.
2. Bellingham, A. J., Detter, J. C., and Lenfant, C.: Regulatory mechanisms of hemoglobin oxygen affinity in acidosis and alkalosis. J. Clin. Invest., 50:700, 1971.
3. Benesch, R., and Benesch, R. E.: The effect of organic phosphates from the human erythrocyte on the allosteric properties of hemoglobin. Biochem. Biophys. Res. Commun., 26:162, 1967.
4. Berne, R. M., Blackman, J. R., and Gardner, T. H.: Hypoxemia and coronary blood flow. J. Clin. Invest., 36:1101, 1957.
5. Beutler, E., Meul, A., and Wood, L. A.: Depletion and regeneration of 2,3-diphosphoglyceric acid in stored red blood cells. Transfusion, 9:109, 1969.
6. Brewer, G. J., and Eaton, J. W.: Erythrocyte metabolism: Interaction with oxygen transport. Science, 171:1205, 1971.
7. Bunn, H. F., et al.: Hemoglobin function in stored blood. J. Clin. Invest., 48:311, 1969.
8. Canizaro, P. C., Nelson, J., Prager, M. D., and Shires, G. T.: Erythrocyte 2,3-diphosphoglycerate and oxygen delivery following whole blood transfusion. To be published.
9. Chanutin, A., and Curnish, R. R.: Effect of organic and inorganic phosphates on the oxygen equilibrium on human erythrocytes. Arch. Biochem. Biophys., 121:96, 1967.
10. Dawson, R. B., Jr., Dockolaty, W. F., and Gray, J. L.: Hemoglobin function and 2,3-DPG levels of blood stored at 4°C. in ACD and CPD: pH effect. Transfusion, 10:299, 1970.
11. Dawson, R. B., Edinger, M. C., and Ellis, T. J.: Hemoglobin function in stored blood. J. Lab. & Clin. Med., 77:46, 1971.
12. Delivoria-Papadopoulos, M., Roncevic, N. P., and Oski, F. A.: Postnatal changes in oxygen transport of term, premature and sick infants: The role of red cell 2,3-diphosphoglycerate and adult hemoglobin. Pediatr. Res., 5:235, 1971.
13. Duhm, J.: Effects of 2,3-diphosphoglycerate and other organic phosphate compounds on oxygen affinity and intracellular pH of human erythrocytes. Pfluegers Arch., 326:341, 1971.
14. Duhm, J., Deuticke, B., and Gerlach, E.: Complete restoration of oxygen transport function and 2,3-diphosphoglycerate concentration in stored blood. Transfusion, 11:147, 1971.
15. Duhm, J., and Gerlach, E.: On the mechanisms of the hypoxia-induced increase of 2,3-diphosphoglycerate in erythrocytes. Pfluegers Arch., 326:254, 1971.
16. Haidas, S., Labie, D., and Kaplan, J. C.: 2,3-Diphosphoglycerate content and oxygen affinity as a function of red cell age in normal individuals. Blood, 38:463, 1971.
17. Lenfant, C., et al.: Effects of altitude on oxygen binding by hemoglobin and on organic phosphate levels. J. Clin. Invest., 47:2652, 1968.
18. Lenfant, C., Ways, P., and Aucutt, C.: Effect of chronic hypoxic hypoxia on the O_2-

Hb dissociation curve and respiratory gas transport in man. Resp. Physiol., 7:7, 1969.

19. McConn, R., and Del Guercio, L. R. M.: Respiratory function of blood in the acutely ill patients and the effect of steroids. Ann. Surg., 174:436, 1971.

20. Metcalfe, J., et al.: Decreased affinity of blood for oxygen in patients with low-output heart failure. Circ. Res., 25:47, 1969.

21. Morse, M., Cassels, D. E., and Holder, M.: The position of the oxygen dissociation curve of the blood in cyanotic congenital heart disease. J. Clin. Invest., 29:1098, 1950.

22. Naeraa, N., et al.: pH and molecular CO_2 components of the Bohr effect in human blood. Scand. J. Clin. Lab. Invest., 18:96, 1966.

23. Opitz, E., and Schneider, M.: Über die Sauerstoffversorgung des Gehirns und den Mechanismus von Mangelverhungerung. Ergebn. Physiol., 46:126, 1950.

24. Oski, F. A., and Delivoria-Papadopoulos, M.: The red cell, 2,3-diphosphoglycerate, and tissue oxygen release. J. Pediatrics, 77:941, 1970.

25. Oski, F. A., et al.: The in vitro restoration of red cell 2,3-diphosphoglycerate levels in banked blood. Blood, 37:52, 1971.

26. Plzak, L. F., Watkins, G., and Sheldon, G.: Hyperalimentation and the Oxy-Hemoglobin Dissociation Curve. In: G. Cowan and W. Scheety (Editors): Intravenous Hyperalimentation. Philadelphia, Lea & Febiger, 1972.

27. Pollock, T. W., et al.: In vivo effect of inosine, pyruvate, and phosphate (IPP) on oxygen-hemoglobin affinity. Fed. Proc., 30:546, 1971.

28. Roughton, F. J. W.: Some recent work on the interactions of oxygen, carbon dioxide and haemoglobin. Biochemistry, 177:801, 1970.

29. Severinghaus, J. W.: Blood gas calculator. J. Appl. Physiol., 21:1108, 1966.

30. Shafer, A. W., et al.: 2,3-Diphosphoglycerate in red cells stored in acid-citrate-dextrose and citrate-phosphate-dextrose: Implications regarding delivery of oxygen. J. Lab. Clin. Med., 77:430, 1971.

31. Shappell, S. D., and Lenfant, C. J. M.: Adaptive, genetic, and iatrogenic alterations of the oxyhemoglobin-dissociation curve. Anesthesiology, 37:127, 1972.

32. Snyder, L. M., and Reddy, W. J.: Mechanism of action of thyroid hormones on erythrocyte 2,3-diphosphoglyceric acid synthesis. J. Clin. Invest., 49:1993, 1970.

33. Sullivan, S. F.: Oxygen transport. Anesthesiology, 37:140, 1972.

34. Torrance, J., et al.: Intraerythrocyte adaptation to anemia. New Engl. J. Med., 283:165, 1970.

35. Valeri, C. R.: Viability and function of preserved red cells. New Engl. J. Med., 284:81, 1971.

36. Valeri, C. R., and Fortier, N. L.: Red cell 2,3-diphosphoglycerate and creatine levels in patients with red cell mass deficits or with cardio-pulmonary insufficiency. New Engl. J. Med., 281:1452, 1969.

37. Valeri, C. R., and Fortier, N. L.: Red Cell 2,3-DPG, ATP, and Creatine Levels in Preserved Red Cells and in Patients with Red Cell Mass Deficits or with Cardiopulmonary Insufficiency. In: George J. Brewer (Editor): Red Cell Metabolism and Function. New York, Plenum Press, 1970, p. 289.

38. Valeri, C. R., and Hirsch, N. M.: Restoration in vivo of erythrocyte adenosine triphosphate, 2,3-diphosphoglycerate, potassium ion, and sodium ion concentrations following the transfusion of acid-citrate-dextrose-stored human red blood cells. J. Lab. Clin. Med., 73:722, 1969.

39. Wood, L., and Beutler, E.: Storage of erythrocytes in artificial media. Transfusion, 11:123, 1971.

40. Woodson, R. D., et al.: The effect of cardiac diseases on hemoglobin-oxygen binding. J. Clin. Invest., 49:1349, 1970.

Therapy of Shock

Chapter Six

HYPOVOLEMIC SHOCK

It is apparent from the previously described etiologic classification of shock that therapy will of necessity depend on detection of the causative mechanisms, while support of the patient is supplied. Correction of the underlying causative factors can then be carried out. Consequently one sees again the usefulness of a practical clinical classification that includes (1) oligemic shock, (2) cardiogenic shock, and (3) shock caused by changes in peripheral resistance and capacitance vessels (neurogenic shock and septic shock). In a patient who has undergone trauma more than one causative factor may be operating. Once the diagnosis of shock has been made and supportive therapy begun, a deligent search for the causative factor or factors can be made.

Treatment of shock, therefore, can best be thought of in relation to the type of shock that is present. As pointed out earlier, the pathogenesis of hypovolemic hypotension is varied. Recognition of deficits of total body water and electrolytes is usually subtle, and correction requires specific therapy with crystalloid solutions. Reductions in the extracellular fluid volume (plasma and interstitial fluids) primarily, such as in burns, peritonitis and some forms of crush injury, are more easily recognized. Specific therapy should be started with electrolyte solutions and rarely may require the use of plasma or some source of protein. External blood loss as seen in lacerations should be corrected immediately, as fluid therapy is begun, with first-aid measures, including pressure tamponade. Surgical procedures may then be carried out. Similarly, an external loss, such as bleeding from a duodenal ulcer, should be treated with the usual measures, including decompression of the stomach, while supportive therapy is begun.

The only other immediate concern in addition to control of the

119

causative wounds is maintenance of an open airway. Pulmonary insufficiency rarely occurs from shock alone, but concomitant injuries may include crush injuries of the chest, pneumothorax, hemothorax or specific obstruction of the airway from injuries to the head and neck. In these circumstances adequate respiratory exchange must be restored promptly.

VOLUME

The treatment of hemorrhagic shock continues to be the adequate replacement of whole blood, since this is the fluid that has been lost. Early use of properly cross-matched, type-specific whole blood is still the primary therapy when shock is due to whole blood loss. When whole blood of the proper type and crossmatch is not immediately available, type-specific or Rh-negative "universal donor" type O blood with low anti-A titer can be administered.

Extracellular Fluid Replacement

In view of the previously described changes in the peripheral circulation and interstitial fluid, an effective therapeutic regimen for the treatment of hemorrhagic shock has now been used successfully in several thousand patients.

When patients are admitted to the emergency room in hemorrhagic shock, a large-gauge needle or catheter is inserted into an appropriate vein (preferably in the arm) and an infusion of lactated Ringer's solution is begun immediately. At the same time, blood is drawn for type and crossmatching. The lactated Ringer's solution is run at a rapid rate so that in a period of 45 minutes between 1,000 and 2,000 ml of lactated Ringer's solution has been given intravenously. This approach has several advantages.

1. This is a highly effective therapeutic trial to determine the pre-existing amount of blood loss or the presence of continuing blood loss. It is often observed that blood pressure will return to normal, become stable and remain so in patients with severe hypotension, after infusion of 1 or 2 L of a balanced salt solution. When such a response is correlated with measurements of red blood cell mass, plasma volume and extracellular fluid volume, it has been shown that the pre-existing blood loss was relatively minimal. If blood loss has been minimal and hemorrhage is not continuing, then hemorrhagic hypotension can be alleviated simply by the infusion of a balanced salt solution.

2. If blood loss has been severe or hemorrhage is continuing,

then the elevation of blood pressure and decrease in pulse rate that occur with rapid intravenous infusion of lactated Ringer's solution will usually be transient. When this occurs, whole blood that has been accurately typed and crossmatched is available and can be given immediately. Consequently the initial use of the balanced salt solution allows time for accurate typing and crossmatching.

3. In view of the large, disparate reduction in the extravascular, extracellular fluid as demonstrated in animals and man, it is felt that even though blood is needed, as it is in the majority of patients admitted in hemorrhagic hypovolemia, alleviation of the reduction in functional extracellular fluid is desirable.

4. Lactated Ringer's solution as initial therapy, both from the standpoint of a therapeutic trial and as a therapeutic adjunct, is a procedure that has been found to be effective. This is understandable, since lactated Ringer's solution is isotonic, essentially free from side reactions, and virtually harmless from the standpoint of aggravation of other fluid and electrolyte imbalances that may be present.

Further, it appears that the use of a balanced salt solution in this fashion significantly reduces the requirement of whole blood in the patient with hemorrhagic hypotension. This is true not only from the standpoint of proper hemoglobin and hematocrit concentrations following therapy, but also from the standpoint of prevention of, or recovery from, renal failure.

A concern that Ringer's lactate solution may aggravate the existing lactate acidosis when used to treat patients in shock has been expressed by several investigators, but previous studies in both experimental animals and patients do not support this view.[4,17,38,61] The use of blood plus Ringer's lactate solution to treat hemorrhagic shock in experimental animals results in a more rapid return to normal of lactate, excess lactate and pH than does treatment with return of shed blood alone.[47] Recently, serial determinations of lactate, excess lactate, pH and base excess have been obtained in 52 patients in hemorrhagic shock.[15] All patients received Ringer's lactate solution in addition to whole blood during the period of resuscitation. There was a significant reduction in lactate and excess lactate levels and a return of pH and base excess values toward normal during the period of shock while Ringer's lactate solution was being infused. After resuscitation, all these values rapidly returned to normal levels (Fig. 6–1).

Blood Transfusions

The acceptability for transfusion of blood which has been stored in ACD solution for up to three weeks is based on survival of at least 70 per cent of the cells in the recipient's circulation. During this

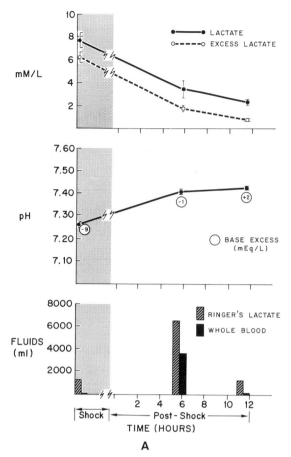

Figure 6–1 A, Mean values (±SE) for 52 patients in hemorrhagic shock. Postshock values are the means of the 48 patients resuscitated from shock. The amount of fluids administered is indicated at the end of each interval.

three-week period, however, there is a rapid decline in erythrocyte 2,3-diphosphoglycerate (DPG) and a progressive increase in hemo-globin-oxygen affinity (leftward shift of the oxygen dissociation curve).[8, 13, 24, 25, 62] After transfusion it requires 24 hours or longer for the DPG levels to return to normal.[14, 64] These findings indicate that oxygen delivery may be impaired after the administration of large quantities of stored blood and have led to a re-evaluation of transfusion practices.

Obtaining a sufficient quantity of fresh blood for resuscitation of the patient in hemorrhagic shock is difficult, and attempts are being made to find a suitable storage medium that will maintain the level of organic phosphates in the red blood cells.[25, 63, 72] At present, storage of blood in CPD (citrate-phosphate-dextrose) solution seems to be the most practical alternative, since DPG is more stable in this medium

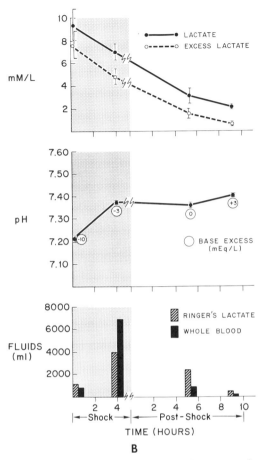

Figure 6–1 Continued. B, Mean values (±SE) for 15 patients who had at least two determinations of lactate and excess lactate during the period of hemorrhagic shock.

than in ACD solution. The administration of limited quantities of older CPD-stored blood in acute situations is acceptable, although the capability of this blood to deliver oxygen fully may not be realized for several hours. When larger quantities of blood are administered, particularly in critically ill patients, the storage age of each unit should be recorded. If a significant portion of the blood administered is more than a few days old, every attempt should be made to obtain fresh blood for additional transfusion requirements.

Consideration of other factors that influence the position of the dissociation curve (Table 5–1, p. 102) may also be important in the individual patient. For instance, the induction of a respiratory alkalosis may produce an abrupt increase in hemoglobin-oxygen affinity. This is a common occurrence during operation and in patients requiring ventilatory assistance in the postoperative period; coupled with other factors that limit oxygen transport, the capacity to maintain tissue oxygenation may be sharply reduced. Similarly, the sudden correction of an acidosis, whether metabolic or respiratory, may have undesirable effects. In this regard the indiscriminate use of sodium bicarbonate during resuscitation of patients in hypovolemic shock is discouraged. The presence of a mild metabolic alkalosis is a common finding after resuscitation, owing in part to the alkalinizing effects of blood transfusions and the administration of lactated Ringer's solution. After infusion (and partial restoration of hepatic blood flow) the citrate and lactate contained in transfused blood and the lactate in lactated Ringer's solution are metabolized and bicarbonate is formed. If excessive quantities of sodium bicarbonate are administered simultaneously, a severe metabolic alkalosis may result. The alkaline pH may be highly undesirable, particularly in patients with hypoxia or low fixed cardiac output. In combination with other factors incident to blood replacement which increase hemoglobin-oxygen affinity (low DPG concentration and hypothermia), significant interference with oxygen unloading at the cellular level may occur.

The immediate and direct pH influences on the curve (via the Bohr effect) are eventually offset by reciprocal changes in DPG concentration. There is a lag period, however, of approximately four hours before any change in DPG concentration is noted, and the final level is not reached until 48 hours after induction of acidosis or alkalosis.[7] The fact that the effects of sudden large changes in pH may persist for several hours should be considered during therapy. Correction of a metabolic acidosis, therefore, is properly directed toward correction of the underlying disorder. Bicarbonate therapy may be reserved for the treatment of severe metabolic acidosis, particularly following cardiac arrest, when *partial* correction of pH is essential to restore myocardial function. Similarly, pH correction in more protracted states of metabolic acidosis may be indicated, but should be accomplished slowly (see Oxygen Transport, page 111).

Hematocrit

For many years the belief was held that hemorrhage and shock are separate entities, because hemorrhage was not accompanied by hemoconcentration, though shock was inevitably accompanied by a rise in hematocrit. As shown in Figure 6–2 and as described previously in the pathologic physiology of shock, the hematocrit is not a differentiating factor. The extent of concentration depends on the proportion of red blood cells and plasma lost in the hypovolemic episode, as well as on the compensatory adjustments that the interstitial fluid has been able to make to the intravascular volume reduction.

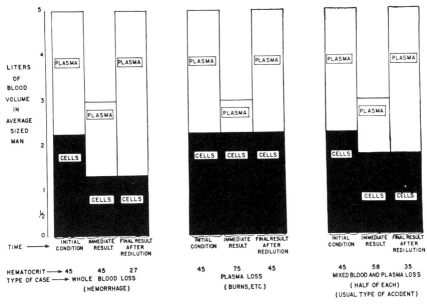

Figure 6–2   Six possible results in shock cases, and the fallacy of using hemoconcentration as the only guide to treatment. (From Harkins, H. N.: Recent advances in the study and management of traumatic shock. Surgery, 9:231–294, 1941.

Blood Substitutes

In the absence of whole blood, many substances have been proposed as transient substitutes for the combination of red blood cells and plasma available in whole blood. The most popular and commonly used substitute has been human plasma. In some circumstances, e.g., battlefield conditions, plasma has been a highly serviceable substitute. Plasma carries with it the same risk of viral hepatitis that whole blood does.[1] A unit of pooled plasma, however, carries a greater risk of harboring and transmitting the infective viral hepatitis than a unit of blood. As shown by Allen, storage of fresh plasma at room temperature for six to eight months significantly reduces the attack rate and infectivity of the virus of infectious hepatitis.[1] In any event, the administration of plasma carries with it some risk of hepatitis as well as the poorly understood antigen-antibody reactions that frequently occur from homologous plasma. Further, the volume of plasma required is such that for all practical purposes restoration of blood volume is not generally feasible with plasma alone. Plasma contains no hemoglobin and, therefore, no oxygen-carrying capacity beyond that of any nonerythrocyte-containing liquid (physically dissolved oxygen in plasma constitutes only 0.3 per cent by volume).

It should be pointed out that volume replacement with plasma is rapidly equilibrated into the total extracellular fluid. The albumin that remains in the vascular tree is easily degraded at a rapid rate. Moore estimates that plasma dispersal from the intravascular to extravascular phase may proceed at a rate approaching 500 ml, or 2 units per hour.[48] Therefore plasma or albumin as a blood volume substitute is transient at best.

A number of other substances have been proposed for transfusion in hemorrhagic shock since early in World War I, when solutions of acacia were used. Several excellent review articles are available which summarize the problems with all these artificial solutions.[29] Suffice it to say that at present the only acceptable one of the entire group continues to be dextran. This substance has been shown to be effective clinically in the absence of a severe need for hemoglobin and its oxygen-carrying capacity. Nevertheless, like all other plasma or blood substitutes, this substance still causes occasional severe antigen-antibody reactions and, above all, regularly produces defects in the clotting mechanism. This has been shown in volunteers and patients when amounts greater than 1 L of clinical dextran with an average molecular weight of approximately 75,000 are used in man.[35] The longest effect of dextran in maintaining an expanded plasma volume has been shown to be 24 to 48 hours. Low-molecular-weight dextran in the average range of 35,000 to 40,000 has recently received renewed interest because of data suggesting its ability to lower the viscosity of blood and possibly to prevent agglutination of erythrocytes during the low-flow state induced by hypovolemic shock.[3, 30, 43] But work by Replogle indicates that the effect of low-molecular-weight dextran on blood viscosity is produced entirely by hemodilution or change in blood volume.[54] When these parameters were controlled, no evidence for alterations in blood viscosity associated with infusions of low-molecular-weight dextran were observed. Although there are some theoretical advantages in using this plasma expander, recent investigative studies are beginning to reveal serious clotting mechanism defects with low-molecular-weight dextran, such as had been seen with the higher-molecular-weight dextrans.

POSITIONING

Positioning of the patient in shock has long been thought to be an adjunct in the treatment of hypovolemic shock. Most first-aid courses teach that the patient in shock should be placed in the head-down position. Although it is true that some forms of shock, particularly neurogenic shock, will respond to the head-down position, the effect of posture on the cerebral circulation in the face of true hypovolemia has not been defined. Frequently the patient with multiple trauma has sustained other injuries, both within the abdomen and the chest, so that the routine use of the Trendelenburg, or head-down, position may interfere with respiratory exchange far more than when the patient is left supine. The beneficial effect of the head-down position is probably the result of transient autotransfusion of pooled blood in the capacitance or venous side of the peripheral circulation. This beneficial effect can be obtained easily by elevating both legs while maintaining the trunk and the remainder of the patient in the supine position. This is probably the preferable position, then, for the treatment of hypovolemic shock.[31]

PULMONARY SUPPORT

In the past most writings on the treatment of hypovolemic shock stated that breathing high oxygen concentrations is probably of little avail during a period of hypotension.[59] These conclusions were based on the concept that the principal defect is in volume flow to tissues and decreased cardiac output. The oxygen saturation in the majority of patients with uncomplicated hypovolemic shock is generally normal, and the small increase in dissolved oxygen in the blood contributed by raising the PO_2 above this level is insignificant, particularly in the face of a markedly decreased cardiac output. This concept continues to be valid in terms of improvement of the shock state or tissue oxygenation itself. Nevertheless, in the small but significant group of patients in hypovolemic shock in whom the oxygen saturation is not normal, the *initial* use of increased oxygen concentrations may be extremely important, since the fall in cardiac output accompanying hemorrhagic shock has been shown to compound existing defects in oxygenation.[51] This may occur in patients with pre-existing defects, such as chronic obstructive lung disease, but more frequently problems in oxygenation arise directly from the patient's injury. Examples of this would be a coexisting pneumothorax, pulmonary contusion, aspiration of gastric contents or blood and larger obstructive problems. Thus, although oxygen is not routinely administered to patients in shock, if any doubt exists as to the possibility of one of these circumstances or as to the adequacy of oxygenation of arterial blood, the initial administration of oxygen until diligent assessment of the injuries to the patient has been made is certainly justified. If oxygen is to be administered to patients under these circumstances, it should be delivered through loose-fitting face masks designed for this purpose. If controlled airway is indicated for other reasons, an endotracheal tube is ideal. The use of nasal catheters, particularly those passed into the nasopharynx, is avoided because of potential complications of pharyngeal lacerations and gastric distention. Gastric rupture has been recorded secondary to such a catheter inadvertently placed into the esophagus. (For a more complete discussion of pulmonary problems associated with shock and injury, see Chapter 4.)

ANTIBIOTICS

Antibiotics were used in the treatment of hypovolemic shock for many years and were thought to exert a protective mechanism against the ravages of hypovolemia. Subsequent data fail to support this hypothesis. The use of antibiotics in patients, however, who have open or potentially contaminated wounds continues to be sound practice, when combined with good surgical débridement and care. Consequently the use of wide-spectrum antibiotics, as well as specific coverage against the streptococcus and staphylococcus, is advisable as a preventive measure in the severely injured patient. Generally, penicillin is used in doses of 1 to 5 million units per 24 hours with parenteral administration of tetracycline in doses of 1 to 2 gm for the first 24 hours. These are started immediately on patients who have sustained hypovolemic shock from trauma.

TREATMENT OF PAIN

Treatment of pain in the patient with hypovolemic shock is rarely a problem from the standpoint of shock itself. If, however, the causative injury produces severe pain as in fracture, peritonitis, injury to the chest wall, and the like, then control of pain becomes mandatory. Generally, when the patient is moved to the emergency facility where physicians and care are available, simple restorative measures, administration of intravenous fluids, passing of catheters, and so forth, will give reassurance. The need for analgesics is greatly reduced, since the need to allay fear and anxiety becomes markedly less. If, however, the patient continues to have severe pain, then the observations made by Henry K. Beecher in World War II become extremely pertinent.[6] Beecher pointed out that many battle casualties received morphine or other narcotic agents by subcutaneous administration early after wounding. Since these analgesics were not put into the circulation immediately, the pain continued and the patient ultimately received several doses that were not absorbed. Once effective therapy was begun for shock, the doses previously administered were absorbed and profound sedation resulted. As a result, the recommendation was made that small doses of narcotics be given *intravenously* for the management of pain in the patient with shock. This has been standard practice for 20 years and relieves pain without contributing significantly to the potentiation of the shock syndrome.

STEROIDS

Adrenal corticoid depletion was commonly regarded as a contributory factor in shock after it was learned that the presence of hypovolemic shock could in itself deplete the adrenal cortex of adrenal cortical steroids. Subsequent studies, however, have shown that adrenal cortical steroid production is stimulated maximally by the presence of hypovolemic shock.[36] Steroid depletion with hypovolemic shock may possibly occur in the elderly patient or in patients who have specific adrenal cortical diseases such as incipient Addison's disease, postadrenalectomy patients, or patients who have had adrenal suppression with exogenous adrenal cortical steroids. In these specific instances the intravenous administration of hydrocortisone is desirable. In the general patient, however, with hypovolemic shock, administration of adrenal corticoids is probably not indicated.[32]

DIGITALIS

Digitalis has been advocated in the treatment of hypovolemic shock. There is no doubt that in some patients, particularly elderly ones, the stress of hypovolemic shock will in itself induce or aggravate cardiac failure. In these patients, digitalis is found to be helpful. Over the years many have investigated the role of the heart as a cause for the irreversible form of hemorrhagic shock, but experimental data obtained in patients indicate that heart failure in response to hypovolemic shock is merely a terminal event. Further evidence of this is supplied by the fact that the central venous pressure does not rise except terminally in hypovolemic shock.[59]

INTRA-ARTERIAL INFUSIONS

Intra-arterial infusions were advocated for many years for the rapid replacement of intravascular volume in hypovolemic hypotension and shock. The weight of evidence at present, supplied by

Hampson, Scott and Gurd,[33] Harkins[34] and others, is that "the side of the circulation into which the blood is transfused is of no importance provided that the same rapid rate can be assured." Consequently the present-day usefulness of intra-arterial transfusion resolves itself to a matter of convenience. If the operative procedure is in the area of a major artery, as in open-chest procedures, then a given quantity of blood may be delivered much faster via the intra-arterial route. Otherwise no specific advantage seems to be offered by the arterial route of transfusion.

HYPOTHERMIA

Since the basic defect during shock is inadequate perfusion to tissues for maintenance of normal metabolism, a logical approach to supportive therapy would include some mechanism to lower the normal tissue metabolism. Hypothermia is available at present to lower metabolism. To be sure, experimental results in animals have demonstrated that induction of hypothermia prior to the onset of hemorrhagic shock will in fact protect against the lethality of the shock.[50] Similarly, some experiments have shown that therapy of hemorrhagic shock with hypothermia has provided some beneficial effect. The available data for evaluation of hypothermia in man with hypovolemic shock are meager. Since the induction of a hypothermic state is a serious undertaking, it is difficult to assess the effects on the severely injured patient. Some available data in man would indicate that under some circumstances, hypothermia may be desirable. These circumstances need to be further elucidated, and are probably concerned with the later stages of prolonged hypovolemic or possibly septic shock.

RENAL HYPOTHERMIA

Local or regional cooling is of proved benefit in protecting the kidney from damage during ischemic periods. The methods of local cooling previously described have been developed in an attempt to reduce postoperative renal complications induced by the total ischemia necessary during renal artery repair, heminephrectomy or stone removal,[21, 57] as well as aorticorenal surgery.[49] Of far more common occurrence are the renal ischemia and resultant renal damage occasioned by hemorrhagic or hypovolemic shock. Since the kidney is rendered ischemic even in mild hypovolemic shock, rapid lowering of intrarenal temperature should afford protection during the prolonged periods of ischemia.[23, 41]

The effective methods of introducing local renal hypothermia previously described are limited for optimal use in emergency situations by requiring (1) the additional operative trauma of mobilization of the kidney; (2) cumbersome, special equipment that is not readily available or is difficult to sterilize and maintain; and (3) careful attention to prevent interference with other operative procedures within the abdominal cavity.[21, 39, 55]

The open peritoneal cavity affords a large surface area for heat exchange. Jaeger found that the introduction of a large volume of cold isotonic solution into the closed peritoneal cavity of dogs resulted in a rapid decrease in body temperature.[37] If intra-abdominal organs, particularly the kidneys, which are apparently the most sensitive to hypoxia, can be effectively cooled by the direct introduction of cold solution, then a simple, expedient, practical method of cooling is readily available in every operating room. This consists in filling the open abdominal cavity with isotonic salt solution that has been cooled in the operating room refrigerator (Fig. 6–3).

Experiments in animals were undertaken (1) to compare the temperatures obtained and the protection afforded the ischemic kidney by this method with that of direct surface hypothermia; (2) to evaluate the depth of cooling obtained in the ischemic versus the intact kidney; and (3) to determine the depth of cooling obtained in the kidney during hemorrhagic shock.[5] A summary of the results of these experiments follows.

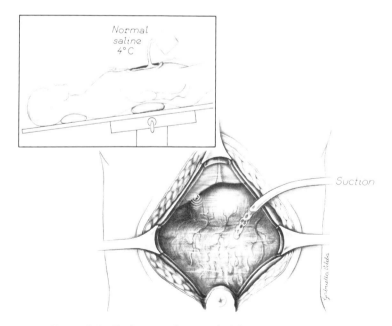

Figure 6–3   Technique of regional abdominal hypothermia.

1. Figure 3–12 (p. 57) shows the degree of protection afforded by surface cooling as opposed to formal hypothermic perfusion. As described on page 57, surface cooling provided significant protection from renal ischemia (100 per cent survival rate). Lower intrarenal temperatures could be obtained by circulating coolant; however, the survival rate was lowered, probably because of the necessary extensive mobilization of the kidney.

2. A subsequent experimental study was designed to evaluate the effect of intact blood supply on the degree of hypothermia obtained by peritoneal cooling. The results of this study are shown in Figure 6–4, and a comparison between esophageal temperatures and renal temperatures with and without intact renal blood supply is also seen. These results demonstrate that there is some decrease in total body temperature, especially with intact blood supply to the kidneys, but that the intrarenal temperature even with intact blood flow is decreased at more than twice the rate of the general body temperature. Without blood flow, the depth of renal hypothermia achieved is three times that of the esophageal temperature as long as cooling is continued. An equally important observation is that the ischemic kidney rewarms only slowly as compared to the kidney with intact blood supply.

3. The results of the third study to determine the depth of cooling obtained during hemorrhagic shock are shown in Figure 6–5. The depth of hypothermia obtained is seen to be approximately the same

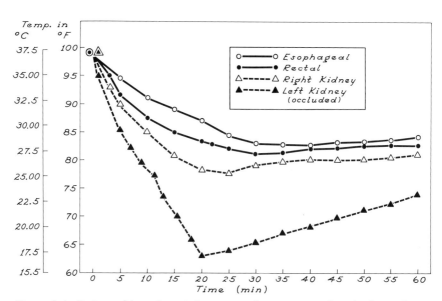

Figure 6–4 Peritoneal hypothermia by means of intraperitoneal iced saline solution at 2–3°C. (left renal pedicle occluded).

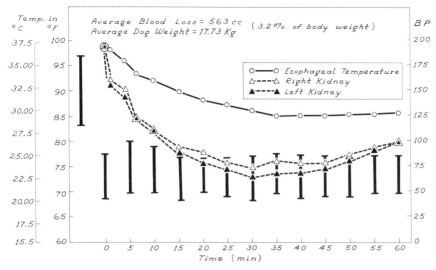

Figure 6–5 Peritoneal hypothermia by means of intraperitoneal iced saline solution at 2–3°C. after blood loss shock (renal pedicle not occluded).

as that in the intact kidneys without hemorrhagic hypotension. Similarly, there was a concomitant lowering of the total body temperature to approximately 88°F. But after the chilled solution had been removed from the abdominal cavity, the intrarenal temperatures in the hypotensive animals continued to decline, reaching 75°F in 30 minutes. Despite this, the total body temperatures did not reach significantly lower levels.

The studies indicate that intrarenal temperatures of approximately 25°C should furnish good protection, with only transient mild suppression of renal function.[11, 40] Certainly 20°C offers complete protection to the ischemic kidney for periods extending to six hours.[12, 27] The effective cooling of the kidney with an intact blood supply versus the ischemic kidney emphasizes the importance of blood supply in determining the rate and depth of cooling.

Studies were then made in patients on the basis of the animal experiments. It was felt that this type of hypothermia could be used in patients with safety, and could be expected to produce a sustained lowering of intrarenal temperatures during hypovolemic hypotension. Intrarenal hypothermia in patients was produced by filling the abdominal cavity with 2 L of refrigerated (3°C) isotonic salt solution. The solution was allowed to remain in contact with the peritoneal cavity for approximately one to two minutes. The bulk of this was removed by suction, and this was repeated several times, employing a total of 4 to 6 L of the cold solution during a five-minute period. Intrarenal temperatures were measured by sterilized needle prior to the induction of hypothermia and at intervals during and after cooling.

Figure 6–6 shows the intrarenal temperatures of 10 patients taken five minutes after the beginning of peritoneal hypothermia. It can be seen that in those patients who were normotensive, there was minimal lowering of the renal temperature. On the other hand, in patients with modest hypotension intrarenal temperatures were lowered to 88 to 90°F, and in the severely hypotensive patient the intrarenal temperature in five minutes had reached the level of 78°F.

Figure 6–7 depicts three patients in whom intrarenal temperatures were measured prior to induction of renal hypothermia and at one-minute intervals thereafter. As would be expected from the studies just presented, the rate of fall of intrarenal temperature was directly proportional to the degree of hypotension present at the time of cooling.

Esophageal temperatures were monitored. In general, the fall in esophageal temperature was approximately half the fall in intrarenal temperatures in the first 10 minutes. The lowest temperature reached was 88°F in two patients. No untoward effects were noted other than a modest fall in blood pressure (less than 10 mm/Hg diastolic) in normotensive patients. There were no changes in cardiac rate or rhythm during this procedure.

The animal experiments show that an intrarenal temperature of 28 to 30°C is easily attainable in the ischemic dog kidney by sluice cooling of the peritoneal cavity. This moderate degree of hypothermia produced 100 per cent survival, but with mild elevation of the BUN

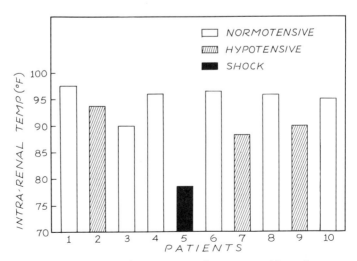

Figure 6–6   Intrarenal temperature after peritoneal hypothermia.

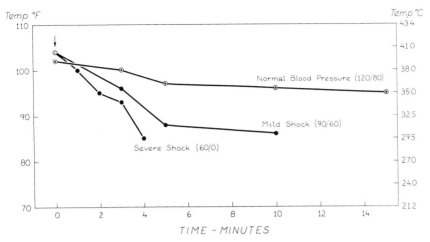

Figure 6–7 Regional hypothermia in patients.

for a period of 12 to 15 days. All these animals excreted normal or increased amounts of urine.

The preliminary data suggest that cooling by means of peritoneal irrigation (1) produces sufficient lowering of intrarenal temperatures to afford protection to the kidney with decreased blood flow; (2) offers a rapid means of lowering total body temperature; and (3) should produce a decrease in intrarenal temperature in a kidney completely deprived of blood comparable to that obtained by other local techniques.

In the past the chief objection to peritoneal irrigation was the introduction of infection. Peritoneal dialysis for uremia has proved to be a safe procedure on a short-term basis, infection occurring only after prolonged use.[26] In our experience the use of copious quantities of refrigerated salt solution in the operating room has been completely free from complications. Specifically, there have been no cases of peritonitis, abscess formation, wound disruption or prolonged ileus in the patients studied.

VASOPRESSORS

In recent years the addition of substances that cause additional vasoconstriction in hypovolemic shock has been popular. These have largely been used because the blood pressure in man can usually be elevated somewhat by the addition of one of a series of pressor agents. Although it is true that blood pressure can be elevated, the objective in treating hypovolemic shock is one of increasing tissue perfusion. By use of vasopressors the blood pressure is raised by increasing peripheral vascular resistance and decreasing tissue perfusion. Therefore the injurious effects of shock may well be aggravated.

As experience has accumulated with the use of vasopressors, it is obvious that the alpha and beta stimulating functions of the vasopressors must be separated during clinical evaluation (Fig. 6–8).[44] The vasopressors generally have a threefold action consisting of central inotropic and chronotropic effects, as well as a peripheral vasoconstricting effect. In a recent evaluation of the comparative effects of a number of the catecholamines, Waldhausen et al. demonstrated significant differences.[65] Isoproterenol hydrochloride (Isuprel), levarterenol bitartrate (Levophed), epinephrine (Adrenalin) and phenylephrine hydrochloride (Neo-Synephrine) all produced a significant increase in contractility of the heart and an increase in heart rate. Isoproterenol had, in addition, a vasodilator effect on the peripheral vessels, while the other three amines were largely peripheral vasoconstrictors. Metaraminol (Aramine) produced a significant increase in myocardial contractility, further increasing the efficiency of the heart beat while the heart rate fell; this amine was also a moderate vasopressor. Of the drugs tested, phenylephrine showed the least

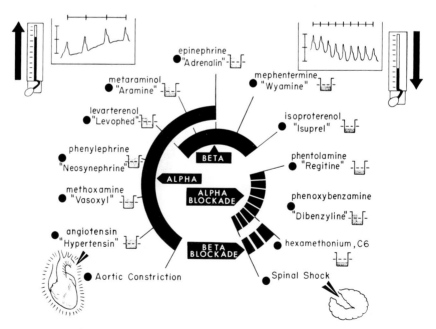

Figure 6–8 Adrenergic mechanisms. (From C. M. Lewis and M. H. Weil: Hemodynamic spectrum of vasopressor and vasodilator drugs. J.A.M.A., *208*:1391, 1969. Copyright, 1969, American Medical Association.)

efficient inotropic effect and was predominantly a peripheral vaso-pressor.

In 1923 Cannon condemned the use of vasopressors on this physi-ologic basis: "Damming the blood in the arterial portion of the cir-culation, when the organism is suffering primarily from a diminished quantity of blood flow, obviously does not improve the volume flow in the capillaries."[16] In 1940 Blalock also condemned the use of vaso-pressors in treating shock.[9] Recent studies have more clearly defined the hazards of using vasopressors in hypovolemic shock. Close and his associates demonstrated a sharp increase in the mortality of dogs rendered hypotensive by hemorrhage when norepinephrine was administered in sufficient doses to raise the blood pressure from 40 mm Hg to 100 mm Hg.[20] Mortality in animals so treated was 64 per cent compared with 33 per cent in the untreated controls. Catchpole et al., using a drip of norepinephrine after 30 minutes of hypotension and again before reinfusion of shed blood, obtained no improvement in survival.[19] Additionally, Hakstian, Hampson and Gurd demon-strated no significant protection during hemorrhagic hypotension through the use of norepinephrine.[32] On the other hand, studies by Lansing and Stevenson suggest that the use of norepinephrine for the maintenance of blood pressure and cardiac output *after* normovole-mia has been restored may be advantageous.[42] Simeone has similarly shown that the use of vasopressors after restoration of normal blood volume may be of some significant help if applied early.[60] Probably the beneficial effects of these experimental studies can be related more properly to their inotropic effect on the heart than to their vaso-constrictor properties. This is especially true since these studies show benefit only after volume has been restored.

There is other available evidence that the administration of vaso-pressors during hypovolemia will reduce the already depleted plasma volume. Our own data would tend to support this concept.[18, 56]

The use of vasopressors in hemorrhagic shock is rapidly disap-pearing. Suffice it to say, as more and more data have become avail-able, it is doubtful whether the use of vasopressors in the treatment of hypovolemic shock is ever warranted.

VASODILATORS

In 1948 Wiggers and his associates predicted that a significantly increased survival rate in animals treated with an adrenergic blocking agent and subjected to hemorrhagic shock would indicate the detri-mental influence of protracted vasoconstriction in shock.[68] Subse-quently, in 1950, Remington and his associates reported an increased survival rate in dogs pretreated with Dibenamine before the induction of hemorrhagic shock.[53] Zweifach, Baes and Shorr[73] similarly found that Dibenamine protected rats against lethal graded hemorrhage if the animals were pretreated, and Boba and Converse[10] reported that ganglionic blocking agents increased the survival of experimentally shocked animals.

Webb et al. found that the administration of hydralazine during the hypovolemic hypotensive phase of experimental hemorrhagic shock was deleterious. [6] In contrast, Hakstian, Hampson and Gurd obtained 15 survivals out of 16 animals subjected to hemorrhagic shock and treated with hydralazine during the shock period.[32] Collins, Jaffee and Zahony reported survival in a study of 396 patients treated with chlorpromazine; 186 of these patients were treated after the onset of shock, and the survival rate was said to be twice that of the control group.[22] Longerbeam, Lillehei and Scott found that giving Dibenzyline (phenoxybenzamine) led to a remarkable improvement in the mortality rate of their animals.[45] Thal recently reported encouraging results with Dibenzyline in the treatment of refractory normovolemic endotoxic shock.[71]

HEMODYNAMIC MEASUREMENTS

A patient in hemorrhagic or oligemic shock may rarely fail to respond to vigorous management as outlined above. Such a patient usually presents a complicated clinical picture. Frequently surgical procedures have been carried out for correction of the underlying causes of shock. Thus the problem is often compounded by massive fluid and blood administration, general anesthesia and surgical trauma. At this point a comprehensive but rapid re-evaluation of the patient must be carried out in order to institute effective therapy.

The basic defect underlying this "refractory shock" must be corrected. Possible causes are multiple: (1) continuing blood loss from the primary injury or disease or from another source must always be considered; (2) inadequate replacement of fluids; (3) massive trauma, and other derangements secondary to the trauma must be considered, especially cardiac tamponade and pneumothorax; (4) myocardial insufficiency either as a direct result of inadequate perfusion for a prolonged period or secondary to anesthetic agents may be present; and (5) even concomitant septic shock, as with intraperitoneal contamination from bowel perforation, may be a significant factor. The answer to this problem can best be obtained from careful clinical evaluation of the patient and evaluation of a few relatively simple hemodynamic parameters that may serve as a guide to satisfactory treatment.

Clinical evaluation includes a search for signs of bleeding, detection and correction of metabolic abnormalities, and re-evaluation of the primary cause. Special attention must be paid to the adequacy of ventilation, with control of the airway and use of assisted respiration when necessary. In patients who have undergone prolonged surgical procedures requiring the use of a muscle relaxant, subtle hypoventilation can be a significant problem.[58]

In order to be of value, hemodynamic measurements should include an evaluation of several parameters. First, some estimate of the amount of fluid available for circulation is imperative. Second, the ability of the cardiovascular system to circulate this fluid adequately must be evaluated. This includes an evaluation of the efficacy of the heart and of the resistance of the vascular system.

With reference to the amount of fluid available for pumping, direct measurement of the blood volume initially seemed to be the appropriate approach; however, for several reasons, acute blood volume measurements have proved to be unreliable as a guide for therapy of hemorrhagic shock.[67] If the plasma volume alone is measured, an estimate of the total blood volume requires the use of the hematocrit for calculation. These estimated volumes are no more reliable than the hematocrit itself, which has been established to be erratic in hemorrhagic shock. Furthermore, the anatomic blood volume has little relation to that available for circulation if a large portion of this is involved at the site of injury or inflammation or trapped in some vascular pool.

Determination of the extracellular fluid volume would seem extremely useful; however, this remains largely a research tool, since a rapid bedside method is not practical. Use of central venous pressure monitoring has recently been popularized.[70] This technique can be performed easily, and measurements can be repeated often. The central venous pressure has been shown to be a relatively reliable approximation of the efficacy of venous return. The information gained by this method is enhanced if the venous pressure response to the rapid administration of fluids is assessed.[69]

The second of the two parameters requires evaluation of arterial blood pressure by either cuff or arterial cannulation, and some estimate of cardiac output. Cardiac output can be estimated by using arteriovenous oxygen difference as described by Wilson;[69] however, more rapid and direct measurements of cardiac output by the dye dilution principle are now available. These require only intra-arterial cannulation in addition to the central venous catheter, and seem justified in these few critically ill patients.

With the use of these measurements the best method for treatment of the patient's hypotension can frequently be ferreted out of a complicated clinical picture. A depressed or normal central venous pressure that does not rise significantly with rapid administration of a balanced salt solution is usually indicative of a continuing hypovolemia. The diagnosis is supported by the presence of a measured decrease in cardiac output. If the hypovolemia is secondary to inadequate fluid replacement, a gradual and sustained rise in arterial pressure and cardiac output will result from the administration of appropriate fluids. If, on the other hand, continued fluid loss or acute bleeding is the cause, then fluid administration will produce either a transient rise or no rise in the blood pressure and cardiac output.

The presence of an elevated central venous pressure or a central venous pressure that rises with the rapid administration of fluids (and produces either no change or a decrease in cardiac output) is indicative of impairment of the pumping mechanism. Usually this represents primary myocardial deficiency and must be treated accordingly; however, the defect in the pumping mechanism may rarely be due to mechanical obstruction as with cardiac tamponade or mediastinal compression by intrapleural fluid or air. The possible presence of these surgically correctable lesions must be kept in mind, especially in the patient who has multiple injuries. Pulmonary embolism can produce a similar response, but is rarely seen early in the course of the injured patient.

A normal or slightly increased central venous pressure with a normal or high cardiac output and disproportionate hypotension is usually due to a loss of peripheral vascular resistance. Decreased peripheral resistance is rarely, if ever, seen in uncomplicated oligemic shock and, if present, should alert one to the possibility of a "septic" component. The converse is usually true in oligemic shock, since peripheral resistance is markedly increased; if accompanied by deficient myocardial function, the use of an inotropic agent (with minimal vasoconstrictor or preferably with vasodilator effects) may be beneficial.[46] This should be done only after more direct measures such as adequate volume replacement or digitalization have been vigorously pursued. Hemodynamic measurements usually fail to show any indication for use of a vasoconstrictive agent in the therapy of hemorrhagic shock.

Several authors have questioned the value of central venous pressure measurements and pointed out that left ventricular overload and pulmonary edema can occur while right ventricular function (and the central venous pressure) remains adequate.[2, 28, 52] This is particularly true after myocardial injury and is discussed more fully in the section on Cardiogenic Shock (p. 146).

In patients with normal cardiac reserve, however, *changes* in the central venous pressure with fluid infusion *do* indicate the ability of the myocardium to pump the volume presented to it. Thus, properly applied, the central venous pressure remains a useful clinical tool. Its interpretation can be augmented by measurement of pulmonary artery pressure when available, but such techniques are usually reserved for patients with more complicated and chronic problems.

The ultimate hemodynamic criterion in the treatment of shock is the response of the patient. Two indications of adequate resuscitation are restoration of adequate cerebration and urine output. Although diuresis by any means may be beneficial when a large pigment load is presented to the kidneys, the object of treatment in hypovolemic shock is to re-establish urine flow by adequate restoration of circulation, and not to force urine flow in spite of inadequate resuscitation. The use of osmotic diuretics in the presence of uncorrected oligemic shock to produce "urine for urine's sake" would seem to have no physiologic basis and may, in fact, be detrimental by further depleting intravascular and extravascular extracellular fluid.

REFERENCES

1. Allen, J. G., Inouye, H. S., and Sykes, C.: Homologous serum jaundice and pooled plasma-attenuating effect of room temperature storage on its virus agent. Ann. Surg., *138*:476, 1953.
2. Azzoli, S. G., Shahinian, T. K., and Cha, C.: Correlation among mean central venous pressure, mean pulmonary wedge pressure, and cardiac output after acute hemorrhage and replacement with Ringer's lactate solution in the dog. Am. J. Surg., *123*:385, 1972.
3. Baker, R. J., et al.: Low molecular weight dextran in surgical shock. Arch. Surg., 89:373, 1964.
4. Baue, A. E., Tragus, E. T., Wolfson, S. K., Jr., Cary, A. L., and Parkins, W. M.: Hemodynamic and metabolic effects of Ringer's lactate solution in hemorrhagic shock. Ann. Surg., *166*:29, 1967.
5. Baxter, C. R., et al.: A practical method of renal hypothermia. J. Trauma, 3:349, 1963.
6. Beecher, H. K.: Preparation of battle casualties for surgery. Ann. Surg., *121*:769, 1945.
7. Bellingham, A. J., Detter, J. C., and Lenfant, C.: Regulatory mechanisms of hemoglobin oxygen affinity in acidosis and alkalosis. J. Clin. Invest., *50*:700, 1971.
8. Beutler, E., Meul, A., and Wood, L. A.: Depletion and regeneration of 2,3-diphosphoglyceric acid in stored red blood cells. Transfusion, 9:109, 1969.
9. Blalock, A.: Principles of Surgical Care, Shock and Other Problems. St. Louis, C. V. Mosby Company, 1940.
10. Boba, A., and Converse, J. G.: Ganglionic blockage and its protective action in hemorrhage. Anesthesiology, *18*:559, 1957.
11. Bogardous, G. M., and Schlosser, R. J.: Influence of temperature upon ischemic renal damage. Surg., *39*:970, 1956.
12. Bounous, G., Schumacker, H. B., Jr., King, H.: Studies in renal blood flow: I. Some general considerations. Ann. Surg., *151*:47, 1960.
13. Bunn, H. F., et al.: Hemoglobin function in stored blood. J. Clin. Invest., *48*:311, 1969.
14. Canizaro, P. C., Nelson, J., Prager, M. D., and Shires, G. T.: Erythrocyte 2,3-diphosphoglycerate and oxygen delivery following whole blood transfusion. To be published.

15. Canizaro, P. C., Prager, M. D., and Shires, G. T.: The infusion of Ringer's lactate solution during shock: Changes in lactate, excess lactate and pH. Amer. J. Surg., 122:494, 1971.
16. Cannon, W. B.: Traumatic Shock. New York, Appleton-Century-Crofts, Inc., 1923.
17. Carey, L. C., Lowery, B. D., and Cloutier, C. T.: Hemorrhagic Shock. Curr. Prob. Surg., Jan. 1971.
18. Carrico, C. J., Crenshaw, C. A., and Shires, T.: Effect of vasomotor drugs on the extracellular fluid volume during hemorrhagic shock. Clin. Res., 10:288, 1962.
19. Catchpole, B. N., Hackel, D. B., and Simeone, F. A.: Coronary and peripheral blood flow in experimental hemorrhagic hypotension treated with L-norepinephrine. Ann. Surg., 143:372, 1955.
20. Close, S. A., et al.: The effect of norepinephrine on survival in experimental acute hypotension. Surg. Forum, 8:22, 1957.
21. Cockett, A. T. K.: The kidney and regional hypothermia. Surgery, 50:904, 1961.
22. Collins, V. J., Jaffee, R., and Zahony, I.: Shock, a different approach to therapy. Illinois M. J., 122:350, 1962.
23. Corcoran, A. C., Taylor, R. D., and Page, I. H.: Immediate effects on renal function of the onset of shock due to partially occluding limb tourniquets. Ann. Surg., 148:156, 1957.
24. Dawson, R. B., Jr., Dockolaty, W. F., and Gray, J. L.: Hemoglobin function and 2,3-DPG levels of blood stored at 4C. in ACD and CPD: pH effect. Transfusion, 10:299, 1970.
25. Dawson, R. B., Edinger, M. C., and Ellis, T. J.: Hemoglobin function in stored blood. J. Lab. Clin. Med., 77:46, 1971.
26. Doolan, P. D., et al.: An evaluation of intermittent peritoneal lavage. Am. J. Med., 26:831, 1959.
27. Fohrman, F. A.: Oxygen Consumption of Mammalian Tissue at Reduced Temperatures. Physiology of Induced Hypothermia. Proceedings of a Symposium. Washington, D.C., National Academy of Sciences Research Council, 1956.
28. Forrester, J. S., Diamond, G., McHugh, T. J., and Swan, H. J. C.: Filling pressures in the right and left sides of the heart in acute myocardial infarction. A reappraisal of central-venous pressure monitoring. New Engl. J. Med., 285:190, 1971.
29. Gelin, L. E.: Fluid Substitution in Shock. Shock: Pathogenesis and Therapy, An International Symposium. Stockholm, Academic Press, Inc., 1962.
30. Greenfield, L., and Blalock, A.: Effect of low molecular weight dextran on survival following hemorrhagic shock. Surgery, 55:684, 1964.
31. Guntheroth, W. G., Abel, F. L., and Mullins, G. L.: The effect of trendelenburg's position on blood pressure and carotid blood flow. Surg., Gynec. & Obstet., 119:345, 1964.
32. Hakstian, R. W., Hampson, L. G., and Gurd, F. N.: Pharmacological agents in experimental hemorrhagic shock. Arch. Surg., 83:335, 1961.
33. Hampson, L. G., Scott, H. J., and Gurd, F. N.: A comparison of intraarterial and intravenous transfusion in normal dogs and in dogs with experimental myocardial infarction. Ann. Surg., 140:56, 1954.
34. Harkins, H. N.: Shock, Surgery: Principles and Practice. Philadelphia, J. B. Lippincott Company, 1961, pp. 104–125.
35. Howard, J. M., et al.: Studies of dextrans of various molecular sizes. Ann. Surg., 143:369, 1956.
36. Hume, D.: Discussion of Some Neurohumoral and Endocrin Aspects of Shock. Fed. Proc. Supp. No. 9, pp. 87–97, 1961.
37. Jaeger, H. W.: Panel Discussion on the Advantages and Disadvantages of Various Methods in Hypothermia. International Symposium on Cardiovascular Surgery. Philadelphia, W. B. Saunders Company, 1955.
38. James, P. M., Bredenberg, C. E., Anderson, R. N., and Hardaway, R. M.: Tolerance to long and short term lactate infusion in men with battle casualties subjected to hemorrhagic shock. Surg. Forum, 20:543, 1969.
39. Jones, W. R., and Politano, V. A.: Acute renal ischemia and regional renal hypothermia. Surg. Forum, 13:497, 1962.
40. Karr, W. K., et al.: Renal hypothermia. J. Urol., 84:236, 1960.

41. Lamport, H., in Fulton, J. F. (Ed.): Howell's Textbook of Physiology. 16th ed. Philadelphia, W. B. Saunders Company, 1949, p. 580.
42. Lansing, A. M., and Stevenson, J. A. F.: Mechanisms of action of norepinephrine in hemorrhagic shock. Amer. J. Physiol., *193*:289, 1958.
43. Lepley, D., Jr., et al.: Effect of low molecular weight dextran on hemorrhagic shock. Surgery, *54*:93, 1963.
44. Lewis, C. M., and Weil, M. H.: Hemodynamic spectrum of vasopressor and vasodilator drugs. JAMA, *208*:1391–1398, 1969.
45. Longerbeam, J. K., Lillehei, R. C., and Scott, W. R.: The nature of hemorrhagic shock; A hemodynamic study. Surg. Forum, 8:1, 1962.
46. MacLean, L. D., et al.: Treatment of shock in man based on hemodynamic diagnosis. Surg., Gynec. & Obstet., *120*:1, 1965.
47. McClelland, R. N., Shires, G. T., Baxter, C. R., Coln, C. D., and Carrico, J.: Balanced salt solution in the treatment of hemorrhagic shock. JAMA, *199*:830, 1967.
48. Moore, F. D.: The effects of hemorrhage in body composition. New Eng. J. Med., *273*:567, 1965.
49. Moyer, J. H., et al.: Hypothermia. III. Effect of hypothermia on renal damage resulting from ischemia. Ann. Surg., *148*:156, 1957.
50. Overton, R. C., and DeBakey, M. D.: Experimental observations on the influences of hypothermia and autonomic blocking agents on hemorrhagic shock. Ann. Surg., *143*:439, 1956.
51. Pontoppidan, H., Laver, M. B., and Geffin, B.: Acute Respiratory Failure in the Surgical Patient. In: Advances in Surgery, Vol. 4 (Ed. by C. Welch). Chicago, Year Book Medical Publishers, 1970.
52. Rahimtoola, S. H., et al.: Relationship of pulmonary artery to left ventricular diastolic pressures in acute myocardial infarction. Circulation, *46*:283, 1972.
53. Remington, J. W., et al.: Role of vasoconstriction in the response of the dog to hemorrhage. Am. J. Physiol., *161*:116, 1950.
54. Replogle, R. L., Kundler, H., and Gross, R. E.: Studies in the hemodynamic importance of blood viscosity. J. Thorac. & Cardiov. Surg., *50*:658, 1965.
55. Schloerb, P. R., Waldorf, R. D., and Welsh, J. S.: The protective effect of kidney hypothermia on total renal ischemia. Surg. Forum, 8:633, 1957.
56. Schmutzer, J. J., Raschke, E., and Maloney, J. V., Jr.: Intravenous *l*-norepinephrine as a cause of reduced plasma volume. Surgery, *50*:452, 1961.
57. Semb, C.: Partial resection of the kidney: Anatomical, physiological and clinical aspects. Ann. Roy. Coll. Surgeons England, *19*:137, 1956.
58. Shires, G. T. (Ed.): Care of the Trauma Patient. New York, McGraw-Hill Book Company, Inc., 1966, Chap. 6.
59. Simeone, F. A.: Shock. In Christopher's Textbook of Surgery. Philadelphia, W. B. Saunders Company, 1964, pp. 58–62.
60. Simeone, F. A., Husni, E. A., and Weidner, M. G., Jr.: The effect of *l*-norepinephrine upon the myocardial oxygen tension and survival in acute hemorrhagic hypotension. Surgery, *44*:168, 1958.
61. Trinkle, J. K., Rush, B. F., and Eiseman, B.: Metabolism of lactate following major blood loss. Surgery, *63*:782, 1968.
62. Valeri, C. R.: Viability and function of preserved red cells. New Eng. J. Med., *284*:81, 1971.
63. Valeri, C. R., and Fortier, N. L.: Red Cell 2,3-DPG, ATP, and Creatine Levels in Preserved Red Cells and in Patients with Red Cell Mass Deficits or with Cardiopulmonary Insufficiency. In: Red Cell Metabolism and Function, Ed. by George J. Brewer, New York, Plenum Press, 1970, p. 289.
64. Valeri, C. R., and Hirsch, N. M.: Restoration *in vivo* of erythrocyte adenosine triphosphate, 2,3-diphosphoglycerate, potassium ion, and sodium ion concentrations following the transfusion of acid-citrate-dextrose-stored human red blood cells. J. Lab. Clin. Med., *73*:722, 1969.
65. Waldhausen, J. A., Kilman, J. W., and Abel, F. L.: Effects of catecholamines on the heart. Arch. Surg., *91*:86, 1965.
66. Webb, W. R., Shahbazi, N., and Jackson, J.: Metabolic effects of vasopressors and

vasodilators in the hypovolemia of standard hemorrhagic shock. Surg. Forum, *10*:378, 1960.
67. Welch, C. E. (Ed.):ᴗBlood Volume Measurement: A Critical Study. In: F. J. Dagher, et al.: Advances in Surgery. Chicago, Year Book Medical Publishers, Inc., 1965.
68. Wiggers, H. C., et al.: Vasoconstriction and the development of irreversible hemorrhagic shock. Am. J. Physiol., *153*:511, 1948.
69. Wilson, J. N.: Rational approach to management of clinical shock. Arch. Surg., *91*:92, 1965.
70. Wilson, J. N., et al.: Central venous pressure in optimal blood volume maintenance. Arch. Surg., *85*:563, 1962.
71. Wilson, R. F., Jablonski, D. V., and Thal, A. P.: The usage of dibenzyline in clinical shock. Surgery, *56*:172, 1964.
72. Wood, L., and Beutler, E.: Storage of erythrocytes in artificial media. Transfusion, *11*:123, 1971.
73. Zweifach, B. W., Baes, S., and Shorr, E.: Effect of dibenamine against the fatal outcome of hemorrhagic and traumatic shock in rats. Fed. Proc., *11*:7, 1952.

Chapter Seven

CARDIOGENIC, NEUROGENIC, AND SEPTIC SHOCK

CARDIOGENIC SHOCK

In this form of shock the heart fails as a pump. Consequently primary therapy is directed toward the heart. Cardiac arrythmias, whatever their origin, should be treated promptly. Cardiac tamponade, if this is the cause, should be relieved by pericardiocentesis. When the origin of the pump failure is myocardial infarction or myocarditis, then the primary therapy again is directed toward the myocardial damage. If the myocardial damage is sufficiently severe to produce reduction in blood pressure, and indeed in organ perfusion, to the point that organ functions begin to fall, then drugs with positive inotropic action may be efficacious.

Hemodynamic Measurements

Hemodynamic measurements play an important role in the management of postoperative patients with this type of hypotension. As previously described, the classic findings are a central venous pressure that is elevated or rises briskly with fluid administration. This is accompanied by a cardiac output that is depressed and fails to respond to fluid administration. In evaluating postoperative hypotension, as after an extensive procedure in the elderly or especially after

145

cardiac surgery, the measurement of hemodynamic parameters may be of great benefit in differentiating hypovolemic hypotension from hypotension due to depressed myocardial function.[13, 39, 40]

When hemodynamic measurements suggestive of deficient pumping action are found, myocardial insufficiency is usually at fault. It should be stressed again, however, that this can be due to mechanical obstruction (e.g., cardiac tamponade or mediastinal compression in the injured patient and pulmonary embolism in the postoperative patient), and treatment directed at primary myocardial insufficiency can lead to unnecessary delay and catastrophic results. Although identification of abnormalities causing mechanical obstruction to venous return or myocardial function must rest largely on clinical grounds, hemodynamic measurements may be of some benefit in that one may find a slow increase in cardiac output and arterial blood pressure accompanying the rising venous pressure produced by rapid fluid administration. This is in contrast to the picture usually seen in pure myocardial insufficiency, in which the cardiac output frequently falls in the face of a rising venous pressure. The rise in cardiac output is probably because the rising venous pressure is partially effective in overcoming the obstruction and maintaining a nearer normal cardiac filling.[35]

It has been demonstrated that with myocardial injury and after cardiac surgery, differences in functional reserve of the two ventricles occur and the central venous pressure alone loses a great deal of its reliability.[12, 24, 29, 32] Thus it is in these patients that the use of pulmonary artery pressure, pulmonary wedge pressure and, when feasible, left atrial pressure have their greatest value.[13, 37] Left atrial pressure (or left ventricular end-diastolic pressure) is not necessarily the same as right atrial pressure (or central venous pressure, or right ventricular end-diastolic pressure) under these circumstances.

In patients with low cardiac output from low blood volume who also have certain forms of heart disease, left atrial pressure may be considerably higher than right atrial pressure. Examples of such conditions are mitral stenosis and insufficiency, aortic stenosis and insufficiency, severe hypertension and coronary artery disease. In such patients, unless one is actually measuring left atrial pressure, he should probably stop rapid infusion when right atrial or central venous pressure reaches 12 mm Hg (150 mm saline). The relation between changes in atrial pressure and changes in stroke volume or cardiac output at relatively high atrial pressures is not known. In most patients, however, when atrial pressures are about 15 mm Hg (230 mm saline) further increases do not seem to increase cardiac output. Thus, when central venous or right atrial pressure is less than 6 mm Hg (80 mm saline), augmentation of blood volume is indicated. As the infusion proceeds, if central venous pressure rises rapidly and there is little evidence of increase in cardiac output, the infusion should probably be discontinued as being ineffective.

Abnormalities in Contractility

In the condition in which there is low cardiac output and high atrial pressures, and tamponade and ventricular outflow obstruction have been ruled out, there is probably an acute reduction of myocardial contractility. Treatment must therefore be directed toward improving contractility.[8, 11, 15, 26, 38]

The drugs to be considered are:

1. **Digitalis.** If time permits, digitalis is given, and digoxin is recommended. The estimated digitalizing dose given intravenously to a child or adult is 0.9 mg/M^2 of body surface area (1.5 mg for average adult). Half or two thirds of this may be given initially intravenously. An effect can be seen in 10 to 20 minutes, and its peak effect is reached in about two hours. After one to three hours, if no contraindication develops and further effect is desired, an additional one sixth of the estimated digitalizing dose is given. This may be repeated after another two to three hours. In less acute situations the same drug may be given orally, and the digitalizing dose is then 1 mg/M^2. The estimated daily maintenance dose is one quarter of the estimated digitalizing dose, and is usually given in divided doses.

2. **Catecholamines.** Isoproterenol has a specific ionotrophic effect on cardiac muscle, and theoretically is the drug of choice when one needs a prompt and potent agent. It has also a peripheral vasodilating effect which may produce increased hypotension in a patient in shock. Because of a tendency to produce tachycardia and ventricular irritability, isoproterenol is particularly useful when the pulse rate is slow. It is administered by slow intravenous infusion drop by drop of a solution of 0.5 mg of isoproterenol in 250 ml of 5 per cent glucose in water (2 μgm/ml). The rate of infusion is regulated to obtain the desired hemodynamic effect.

Norepinephrine or epinephrine may be used when undue hypertension results from isoproterenol. They increase systemic venous tone and therefore can increase both right and left atrial pressures strikingly; thus caution is indicated, since pulmonary edema can result. These drugs are given intravenously by drop-by-drop infusion of a solution containing 4 mg in 250 ml of 5 per cent glucose in water. Prior to treating patients with low cardiac output and high atrial pressures with these drugs on the basis that the cause is poor myocardial contractility, one must rule out pericardial tamponade. If high intrapericardial pressure exists in patients with high atrial and ventricular end-diastolic pressure, transmural pressure is low and the poor output is due to end-diastolic ventricular volume and fiber length. The treatment is relief of the pericardial tamponade, which is about the only acute cause of high atrial pressures and small end-diastolic ventricular volume. A clinical analysis and chest x-ray are helpful in establishing the diagnosis. The presence of a paradoxic pulse should suggest strongly the presence of tamponade, and needle aspiration or open pericardiotomy is indicated.

3. Ganglionic Blockade. Some patients with low cardiac output and high atrial pressures have relatively high arterial blood pressure. Systemic arteriolar resistance is high (*afterload-load* resisting shortening of myocardial sarcomeres). In these circumstances systolic left ventricular pressure is relatively high, as is systolic ventricular wall stress. Theoretically, reducing arterial blood pressure and systolic ventricular wall stress increases cardiac output.[9, 18] This can be done with an agent such as Arfonad. One should measure cardiac output before and during this drug administration, and only if a significant increase in cardiac output has accompanied the decrease in arterial blood pressure should the drug be continued. Because of the present uncertainties with the use of this drug (such as the effect on coronary, cerebral, liver and renal blood flow) in this situation, it should be given at present only under special circumstances.

Abnormalities in Rate

1. Rapid ventricular rates (over 150 to 180 beats/min.) are usually deleterious to cardiac output. Ventricular end-diastolic pressure is small because of the short period of ventricular filling with tachycardia, and ventricular extensibility is probably decreased because ventricular relaxation is not complete by the end of the extremely short diastolic period. Both tend to reduce stroke volume more than can be compensated for by the rapid heart rate, and cardiac output falls. If atrial fibrillation is the cardiac mechanism, digoxin is the drug of choice. Atrial flutter is more difficult to treat, but should likewise be treated with digoxin. If no progress has been achieved with the drug after two thirds of the digitalizing dose, consideration should be given to electroversion. Atrial tachycardia and premature atrial contractions as causes of excessively rapid heart rates are more difficult still to treat. A continuous intravenous infusion of a drug with pure peripheral vasoconstrictor properties may be helpful (Aramine, 500 mg in 500 ml of 5 per cent glucose in water).

Premature ventricular contractions may on occasion cause fast ventricular rates. Their tendency to cause ventricular fibrillation is of even greater concern. Potassium chloride may be infused over a 10- to 20-minute period. If this is not effective or if the premature ventricular contractions are frequent, lidocaine (Xylocaine) should be given intravenously in a single injection of 50 mg. If further lidocaine is needed, a solution containing 2 mg/ml of lidocaine can be given continuously. If it is used excessively, central nervous system irritability and depression of myocardial contractility may result. If protection against premature ventricular contractions is needed later, Pronestyl (procainamide hydrochloride) can be given orally in doses of 250 to 500 mg every three hours.[3]

2. *Low output associated with ventricular rates of less than 60 to 70 beats/min.* may occur in patients in whom cardiac performance is impaired. Because the myocardium is impaired, stroke volume cannot increase sufficiently to compensate for the slow rate. Regardless of whether the mechanism is sinus rhythm, atrial fibrillation with slow ventricular rate (too much digitalis or too little potassium) or complete atrioventricular dissociation, electrical pacing of the heart at a rate of 80 to 110 beats/min. is advantageous. If there is a sinus mechanism, atrial pacing is preferred. Otherwise, direct ventricular pacing is indicated.[3]

Mechanical Assistance

Effective support for cardiogenic shock may eventually depend on mechanical assistance. Assistive devices are currently available in several centers. At present their use is restricted to patients who do not respond to more conventional therapy.[27, 30, 36]

NEUROGENIC SHOCK

Neurogenic shock or, by the older classification, "primary shock" is that form of shock which follows serious interference with the balance of vasodilator and vasoconstrictor influences to both arterioles and venules. This is the shock that is seen with clinical "syncope" as with sudden exposure to unpleasant events such as the sight of blood, the hearing of ill tidings or even the sudden onset of pain. Similarly, neurogenic shock is often observed with serious paralysis of vasomotor influences, as in high spinal anesthesia. The reflex interruption of nerve impulses also occurs with acute gastric dilatation.

The clinical picture of neurogenic shock is quite different from that classically seen in oligemic or hypovolemic shock. When the blood pressure may be extremely low, the pulse rate is usually slower than normal and is accompanied by dry, warm and even flushed skin. Measurements made during neurogenic shock indicate a reduction in cardiac output, but this is accompanied by a decrease in resistance of arteriolar vessels as well as a decrease in the venous tone. Consequently there appears to be a normovolemic state with a greatly increased reservoir capacity in both arterioles and venules, thereby inducing a decreased venous return to the right side of the heart and subsequently a reduction in cardiac output.

If neurogenic shock is not corrected, there will eventuate reduction of blood flow to the kidneys and damage to the brain, and subsequently all the ravages of hypovolemic shock appear. Fortunately, treatment of neurogenic shock is usually obvious. Gastric dilatation can be rapidly treated with nasogastric suction. High spinal anesthesia can be treated effectively with a vasopressor such as ephedrine or phenylephrine (Neo-Synephrine), which will increase cardiac output as well as produce peripheral vasoconstriction. With the milder forms of neurogenic shock, such as fainting, simply removing the patient from the stimulus or relieving the pain will in itself be adequate therapy so that the vasoconstrictor nerves may regain the ability to maintain normal arteriolar and venular resistance.

There is rarely a need for a hemodynamic measurement in this usually benign and frequently self-limited form of hypotension. Correction of the underlying deficit usually results in a prompt resumption of normal cardiovascular dynamics. The exception to this occurs when this form of shock results from injury, as with spinal cord transection from trauma. In this instance there may be significant loss of blood and extracellular fluid into the area of injury surrounding the cord and vertebral column. Considerable confusion can arise as to the relative need for fluid replacement, as opposed to the need for vasopressor drugs under these circumstances. Similarly, if surgical intervention for any reason becomes necessary, hemodynamic measurements may be of great value in the management of these patients. In uncomplicated neurogenic shock, central venous pressure should be normal or slightly low with a normal or elevated cardiac output. On the other hand, as hypovolemia ensues, central venous pressure decreases, as does the cardiac output. Thus careful monitoring of the central venous pressure may be of great aid. Fluid administration without vasopressors in this form of hypotension may produce a gradually rising arterial pressure and cardiac output without elevation of central venous pressure, by gradually "filling" the expanded vascular pool; therefore caution must be utilized during fluid administration.

In the management of these patients in balancing the two forms of therapy, slight volume overexpansion is much less deleterious than excessive vasopressor administration. The latter compounds decrease organ perfusion in the presence of inadequate fluid replacement. This balance can best be obtained by maintaining a normal central venous pressure that rises slightly with rapid fluid administration (thus ensuring adequate volume), and using a vasopressor such as phenylephrine judiciously to support arterial pressure.[23]

SEPTIC SHOCK

During the past several years there has been a progressive increase in the incidence of shock secondary to sepsis, and the mortality rate remains in excess of 50 per cent. This has occurred despite a better understanding of this entity, use of newer treatment regimens, and development of more potent antimicrobial agents. The most frequent causative organisms are gram-positive and gram-negative bacteria, although any agent capable of producing infection (including viruses, parasites, fungi and rickettsiae) may initiate septic shock. Because of effective antibiotic control of most gram-positive infections, the majority of septic processes that result in shock are now caused by gram-negative bacteria. Among other causes, Altemeier and associates attribute this rising incidence of gram-negative sepsis to (1) the widespread use of antibiotics with development of a reservoir of virulent and resistant organisms; (2) concentration in hospitals of large numbers of patients with established infections; (3) more extensive operations on elderly and poor-risk patients; (4) an increasing number of patients suffering from severe trauma; and (5) the use of steroids, immunosuppressive and anticancer agents.[2]

Gram-Positive Sepsis and Shock

The shock state may be caused by gram-positive infections (1) that produce massive fluid losses (necrotizing fasciitis) (2) by dissemination of a potent exotoxin without evident bacteremia (Colostridium perfringens and tetani), or (3) most often, by a fulminating infection from staphylococcus, streptococcus or pneumococcus organisms. In the latter instance, shock is theoretically related to the release of exotoxins which many strains of staphylococcus and streptococcus (but not pneumococcus) are known to produce. The hemodynamic changes that occur are different from those seen in shock due to gram-negative organisms. Kwaan and Weil have noted hypotension of comparable severity in shock from both gram-positive and gram-negative infections, but their patients with gram-positive infections failed to show the other clinical manifestations of shock.[19] Arterial resistance fell, but there was little or no reduction in cardiac output even with progressive hypotension. Urine flow was normal, sensorium clear, and perfusion of other organs was not grossly impaired, since neither acidosis nor a significant increase in serum lactic acid concentration appeared.

Treatment consists in the use of appropriate antibiotics, surgical drainage when indicated, and correction of any existing fluid volume deficit. A rapid and favorable response may be anticipated in many patients, and survival is substantially better than with gram-negative infections.

Gram-Negative Sepsis and Shock

Gram-negative sepsis as a cause of shock is a more frequent and difficult problem. The highest incidence occurs during the seventh and eighth decades of life, and the response to treatment depends to a large extent on the age and previous health of the patient. There have been significant advances in the understanding of this entity, although much of the available information is still subject to controversy.

1. Source. The most frequent source of gram-negative infections is the genitourinary system, and almost half of the patients have had an associated operation or instrumentation of the urinary tract.[2] The second most frequent site of origin is the respiratory system, and many of the patients have an associated tracheostomy. Next in frequency is the alimentary system, with diseases such as peritonitis, intra-abdominal abscesses and biliary tract infections; and then diseases of the integumentary system, including burns and soft tissue infections. Indwelling venous catheters for monitoring and hyperalimentation are an increasing source of contamination, particularly with prolonged use. The reproductive system continues to be a significant source of infection (principally from septic abortions and postpartum infections), although the incidence is variable, depending on the hospital population.

The severity of septic shock varies considerably and appears to be a time-dose phenomenon, depending on the type and site of infection. For instance, mild hypotension following instrumentation of the genitourinary tract may represent nothing more than a transient bacteremia which is self-limited or responds to minimal therapy. In contrast, the patient with necrotizing pneumonia or multiple intra-abdominal abscesses may have sepsis from an overwhelming number of organisms for a period of several days, and a much poorer prognosis. Similarly, the outlook is more favorable when the source of infection is accessible to surgical drainage, as in septic abortion, in which the infected products of conception can be removed readily. Variations in these factors must be considered when interpreting reported mortality rates and during the evaluation of new therapeutic regimens.

2. Associated Conditions. The presence of underlying disorders which limit cardiac, pulmonary, hepatic or renal function increases the susceptibility to gram-negative infections and adversely affects the response to treatment. In Altemeier's reported series of 398 patients with gram-negative sepsis, almost half of the patients had a serious associated disease, including diabetes mellitus, malignant neoplasms, uremia, cirrhosis, burns and malignant hematologic disorders.[2] Of these conditions, cirrhosis of the liver appeared to have the most unfavorable prognosis. In addition, a small but significant number of patients were on corticosteroids or immunosuppressive agents, and corresponding mortality rates were 74 and 83 per cent respectively.

3. Bacteriology.   The common causative organisms are similar to those found in the human gastrointestinal tract and include (1) *E. coli;* (2) *Klebsiella aerobacter;* (3) *Proteus;* (4) *Pseudomonas;* and (5) *Bacteroides* in decreasing frequency. Recently the Klebsiella-Enterobacteriaceae-Serratia groups have been isolated with increasing frequency, and many are resistant to more conventional antibiotics.[34] There is also evidence to suggest that Bacteroides species may be the predominant organisms in the fecal flora. These anaerobic organisms are difficult to culture, and may account for a far greater number of infections than was previously reported. The majority of infections are caused by a single gram-negative organism, although in 10 to 20 per cent of cases more than one organism may be isolated.[2, 34] The isolates may be two or more gram-negative organisms or mixed cultures containing both gram-negative and gram-positive bacteria.

4. Clinical Manifestations.   Gram-negative infections are often recognized initially by the development of chills and an elevated temperature above 101°F. The onset of shock may be abrupt and coincident with the signs and symptoms of sepsis or may occur several hours to days after recognition of an established infection. The complex hemodynamic abnormalities that follow are incompletely understood, but are probably initiated by endotoxins from the cell walls of gram-negative bacteria. Intravenous injection of this lipopolysaccharide-protein complex into experimental animals will produce a shock state, but the hemodynamic responses vary in different animal species. The use of experimental animal models has contributed to our understanding of this entity, but direct extrapolation of the findings to human septic shock is difficult. A single injection of endotoxin into dogs causes pooling of blood in the splanchnic circulation, decreased venous return to the heart, reduction in cardiac output and an abrupt fall in blood pressure.[1, 10] This initial response is transient and apparently due to hepatic venous outflow obstruction. Shortly thereafter the blood pressure rises toward normal, but then slowly declines over the next several hours until death of the animal. This pattern is different from that seen in the subhuman primate and in man. Injection of *E. coli.* endotoxin into human volunteers has been shown to produce either (1) no response,[28] (2) chills, fever and vasoconstriction,[28] or (3) peripheral vasodilatation and a rise in cardiac output.[14] These observations emphasize our lack of understanding of the effects of gram-negative infections and septicemia on the human circulation and the need for development of more realistic experimental animal models.

Clinically, the shock state may be characterized by a primary adrenergic response, as seen in hypovolemic shock, with hypotension, peripheral vasoconstriction and cold, clammy extremities. Earlier in the course, however, there may be an absence of adrenergic effects, with warm dry extremities and decreased peripheral resistance. These diverse responses, presumably to the same stimulus, have led to a considerable amount of confusion over the clinical manifestations of septic shock, although a recent report by McLean and associates tends to shed some light on this subject.[21] They have noted two distinct hemodynamic patterns, depending upon the existing volume status of the patient, and believe that the natural history of septic shock is one of progression from respiratory alkalosis to metabolic acidosis. A syndrome of early septic shock occurs in patients who are normovolemic prior to the onset of sepsis and exhibit a hyperdynamic circulatory pattern characterized by (1) hypotension, (2) high cardiac output, (3) normal or increased blood volume, (4) normal or high central venous pressure, (5) low peripheral resistance, (6) warm, dry extremities, (7) hyperventilation, and (8) respiratory alkalosis. A typical patient with this pattern is the young, previously healthy person with a septic abortion. The hemodynamic changes indicate an increased blood flow secondary to peripheral vasodilatation or arteriovenous shunting. In either case the presence of oliguria, altered sensorium and blood lactate accumulation reflect the need for a further increase in flow despite the high cardiac output. McLean suggests that treatment include measures to increase the cardiac output even higher, combined with appropriate antibiotic therapy and early surgical drainage. In his series all but four of 28 patients with this hemodynamic pattern survived the episode of shock. If control of the infection is delayed or unsuccessful, the patient may pass into an acidotic phase with evidence of cellular damage (narrowing arteriovenous oxygen difference, decreasing oxygen consumption) and become refractory to further therapy.

In contrast, if septic shock develops in a patient who is hypovolemic, a hypodynamic pattern emerges characterized by (1) hypotension, (2) low cardiac output, (3) high peripheral resistance, (4) low central venous pressure, and (5) cold, cyanotic extremities. This response is typically seen in a patient with strangulation obstruction of the small bowel and a moderate to severe extracellular fluid and plasma volume deficit. If seen early, these patients are also alkalotic and will respond favorably to treatment. In the absence of overt cardiac failure, prompt volume replacement will often increase cardiac output, and a more favorable hyperdynamic circulation may develop. If therapy to combat sepsis is delayed or unsuccessful, the patient will inevitably have cardiac and circulatory failure with a low fixed cardiac output and a resistant metabolic acidosis. At this point the patient may not be salvageable.

Our own experience in the treatment of septic shock tends to confirm McLean's findings, although the presence of a metabolic acidosis has not necessarily been an ominous finding. We have seen several patients with hypodynamic and hyperdynamic circulatory patterns and metabolic acidosis in the early phase who have responded satisfactorily to therapy. The clinical picture may also be influenced by the patient's ability to meet the increased circulatory requirements imposed by sepsis. The elderly patient with limited cardiac reserve may be unable to increase cardiac output and enter the hyperdynamic phase, even with prompt volume replacement and measures designed to increase cardiac efficiency. In this instance the typical adrenergic response may persist, and the patient may rapidly succumb to the disease process.

Progressive pulmonary insufficiency is characteristically seen in many patients with septic shock. Mild hypoxia with compensatory hyperventilation and respiratory alkalosis are commonly seen early in the course of shock in the absence of clinical or x-ray evidence of pulmonary disease. The arterial desaturation has been attributed to a variety of causes, including the presence of physiologic arteriovenous shunts in the pulmonary circulation secondary to perfusion of atelectatic or nonaerated alveoli (see Progressive Pulmonary Insufficiency, p. 70). Regardless of the cause, the picture is frequently that of rapid deterioration of pulmonary function, development of patchy infiltrates which become confluent, superimposed bacterial infection, severe hypoxemia and death.

Combining all these seemingly contradictory findings into a single unified concept is impossible at present, although Berk has recently suggested that excessive beta adrenergic stimulation is the predominant response in septic shock and causes opening of splanchnic and pulmonary arteriovenous shunts.[5, 6] This would produce a sudden drop in blood pressure and peripheral resistance and a compensatory increase in cardiac output. Shunting of poorly oxygenated pulmonary blood into the arterial circulation would lead to hypoxia, compensatory hyperventilation and respiratory alkalosis. Arteriovenous shunting may also cause increased capillary hydrostatic pressure, stagnant hypoxia of the pulmonary capillaries and a loss of pulmonary surfactant, leading to alveolar collapse and progressive pulmonary consolidation. This attractive hypothesis lacks adequate supportive data, but deserves additional investigation because of its therapeutic implications.

Finally, it is worth emphasizing that development of mild hyperventilation, respiratory alkalosis and an altered sensorium may be the earliest signs of gram-negative infection. This triad may precede the usual signs and symptoms of sepsis by several hours to several days. The exact cause is not known, although the condition is thought to represent a primary response to bacteremia. Early recognition of these findings followed by a prompt search for the source of infection may allow proper diagnosis prior to the onset of shock.

5. Treatment. The only effective way to reduce mortality in septic shock is by prompt recognition and treatment of the associated infection prior to the onset of shock. Once shock occurs, the control of infection by early surgical débridement or drainage and use of appropriate antibiotics represents *definitive* therapy. Other recommended measures, including fluid replacement, steroid administration and the use of vasoactive drugs, represent *adjunctive* forms of therapy, and are useful to prepare the patient prior to surgical intervention or to support the patient until the infectious process is controlled. This point deserves special emphasis, since death of the patient is inevitable if the infection cannot be adequately controlled.

As soon as gram-negative sepsis and shock are apparent, a prompt and thorough search for the source of infection is made while instituting other supportive measures. Because of the multiple complicating factors that may accompany endotoxemia, the patient is preferably treated in an intensive care unit. Careful monitoring of arterial pressure (preferably by a percutaneously inserted radial artery catheter), central venous pressure, urine output and arterial and central venous blood gases may be essential for proper management.

If the infectious process is amenable to drainage, operation is performed as soon as possible after initial stabilization of the patient's condition. In some cases surgical débridement or drainage of the infection must be accomplished before the patient will respond, and may be performed under local or general anesthesia. For example, a patient with ascending cholangitis and shock secondary to sepsis may respond temporarily to supportive treatment. Improvement may be short-lived, however, unless prompt drainage of the biliary tract is accomplished. The importance of surgical drainage is emphasized by the experience of McLean et al. in their treatment of 53 patients. Forty-eight per cent of their patients with infections amenable to surgical drainage survived, while only 23 per cent of those not amenable to surgical treatment survived.[21]

a. ANTIBIOTIC THERAPY. The use of specific antibiotics based on appropriate cultures and sensitivity tests is desirable when possible. The results may not be available for several days, but useful information may be gained from previous wound and blood cultures obtained during an earlier phase of the septic process. Generally, however, antibiotics may be chosen on the basis of the suspected organisms and their previous sensitivity patterns. These patterns are sufficiently diverse to preclude selection of a single antibiotic agent which will be effective against all the potential pathogens.

At present an effective combination of antibiotics in our hospital

population includes the use of cephalothin (6 to 8 gm/day intravenously in four to six divided doses) and gentamycin (1.2 to 1.6 mg/kg
intramuscularly four times daily). These are average adult doses and
should be reduced after initial control of the infection and modified
in any patient with impaired renal function. This combination is
effective against a majority of gram-negative organisms, with the
notable exception of *Bacteroides species.* If presence of these organisms is suspected, an antibiotic of known effectiveness (e.g., clinda-
mycin or Chloromycetin) should be added to the regimen.

When culture and sensitivity reports are available, more specific
antibiotic coverage may be initiated if the infection is not under control. Altemeier and associates reported a mortality rate of 54 per cent
from sepsis in patients receiving inappropriate antibiotics and 28 per
cent when appropriate antibiotics were given.[2]

b. FLUID REPLACEMENT. Prompt correction of pre-existing
fluid deficits is essential. A majority of patients will incur fluid losses
from the disease processes that initiate sepsis and shock. "Third space
losses" with massive sequestration of plasma and extracellular fluid
are characteristic of many surgical conditions, including peritonitis,
burns, strangulation obstruction of the bowel and extensive soft tissue
infections.

The type of fluid used will vary, although most "third space
losses" are properly replaced with a balanced salt solution such as
Ringer's lactate. Blood replacement may be needed, depending on the
hemoglobin and hematocrit levels, and plasma or albumin administration may be specifically indicated in an occasional patient. Although
large quantities of replacement fluids may be required, every attempt
is made to prevent volume overload. In addition to other measures,
including response of the patient noted on frequent clinical observation, continuous monitoring of the central venous pressure may serve
as a valuable guideline for fluid administration. The central venous
pressure catheter may be inserted percutaneously into the subclavian
or internal jugular vein (or by cutdown in an antecubital or the external jugular vein), threaded into the superior vena cava and connected to a saline manometer or other pressure-measuring device.
Properly interpreted, the central venous pressure will give a reliable
estimate of the ability of the right side of the heart to pump the blood
delivered to it. It is best used as an upper limit guide; a rapid increase
in central venous pressure, regardless of the initial level, may indicate
that fluid is being administered too rapidly or that the heart is unable
to handle additional volume. If central venous pressure is below 10
cm of water, fluids may be administered as rapidly as tolerated. If
central venous pressure is above this level, fluids are still administered, but at a slower rate of infusion. The central venous pressure
may fall as blood pressure rises, owing to better perfusion of the cor-

onary arteries and improved myocardial function. An abrupt rise in the central venous pressure or a fall in arterial pressure may indicate inability of the heart to respond, and the use of drugs that increase myocardial performance may be considered.[4]

Many patients will respond favorably to fluid administration combined with prompt control of the infection with a rise in blood pressure, an increase in urine output, warming of the extremities and clearing of the sensorium. In these instances no additional therapy may be indicated.

c. STEROIDS.   The use of pharmacologic doses of corticosteroids in the treatment of septic shock is controversial, but has become a common practice. There is no direct evidence that steroids are beneficial in these cases, although favorable responses with improvement in cardiac, pulmonary and renal functions, and better survival rates have been reported.[25, 31, 33, 41] Large doses of steroids are known to exert a modest inotropic effect on the heart and produce mild peripheral vasodilatation. Although these salutary effects may be desirable, there are other, more potent drugs available with similar actions. Others have suggested that steroids protect the cell and its contents from the effects of endotoxin, e.g. by stabilizing cellular and lysosomal membranes.[17]

Short-term, high-dose steroid therapy is associated with a minimal number of complications and is recommended in most cases that do not respond promptly to other measures. Steroids may be administered concomitant with volume replacement or reserved for use if the response to fluid administration is only temporary or produces a rapid rise in central venous pressure. Many dosage schedules have been recommended, and most stress the need for a large initial dose and cessation of therapy within 48 to 72 hours. Our current regimen is based on guidelines suggested by Lillehei.[25] An initial dose of 15 to 30 mg/kg of body weight of methylprednisolone (or equivalent dose of dexamethasone or hydrocortisone) is given intravenously over a five- to 10-minute period. The same dose may be repeated within two to four hours if the desired effects have not been achieved. If a beneficial response is obtained, additional injections are not given unless the effects are only short-lived. Used in this manner, there is rarely a need for more than two doses.

d. VASOACTIVE DRUGS.   Vasopressor drugs with prominent alpha adrenergic effects are of limited value in treatment of this type of shock, since artificial attempts to maintain blood pressure without regard to flow are potentially harmful. Further, they are probably containdicated in hypovolemic patients with increased peripheral resistance in view of the known deleterious effects of prolonged vasoconstriction. Beneficial effects attributed to these agents are probably due to their inotropic effects on the heart, although better drugs are available for this purpose. Rarely, use of a vasoactive drug with mixed alpha and beta adrenergic effects (e.g. metaraminol) may be indicated in a patient with an elevated cardiac output and pronounced hypotension due to very low peripheral resistance. The increase in resistance (and slight increase in cardiac output) may produce a desired rise in blood pressure and improvement in flow.

Vasodilator drugs such as phenoxybenzamine have enjoyed some popularity, particularly when combined with additional fluid administration. Their use is based in part on improved survival of dogs when vasodilator drugs are given prior to the onset of endotoxic shock.[16, 20] These observations probably represent a specific canine response, and cannot be directly extrapolated to human septic shock. Vasodilator agents have also been used in conjunction with adrenergic agents (for their inotropic effects), but data on their usefulness are limited.[42]

Since the heart is frequently unable to meet the increased circulatory demands of sepsis, the use of isoproterenol (Isuprel) would seem ideal when volume replacement and other measures have failed to restore adequate circulation.[21] Isoproterenol has potent inotropic and chronotropic effects on the heart and produces mild peripheral vasodilation. It is a relatively safe drug, but close observation of the patient is necessary, since severe tachycardia or cardiac arrhythmias may occur, particularly in digitalized patients. One or two milligrams of isoproterenol diluted in 500 cc of 5 per cent dextrose in water may be administered by slow intravenous drip at a rate of 1 to 2 micrograms per minute, depending on the response. The infusion should be slowed or stopped completely if significant tachycardia or cardiac arrhythmias occur. In the absence of arrhythmias, a fall in blood pressure may result from the vasodilation induced by Isuprel and indicates the need for additional volume replacement to maintain cardiac filling pressure. This combination may effectively restore blood flow, even though blood pressure remains less than 100 mm Hg. The response is often temporary, but occasionally the infusion may be continued for two to three days without loss of effect or known deleterious effects.[4]

In summary, a "polypharmacy" approach is discouraged, although proper selection and use of vasoactive drugs may offer the needed support until infection can be controlled or eradicated. If eradication is not possible, response to any of these drugs is only temporary. Determination of cardiac output combined with arterial and central venous measurements can be of great benefit in establishing the nature of the hemodynamic alterations and evaluating responses to therapy.

e. DIGITALIS. Digalitis is not routinely administered in the absence of specific indications. Gram-negative sepsis and shock frequently occur in older patients with congestive failure or may precipitate cardiac failure in patients with limited cardiac reserve. In these instances digitalis can be administered cautiously in full doses, although toxicity may occur if the patient is hypokalemic or receiving isoproterenol.

f. PULMONARY THERAPY. Many patients with sepsis and shock will have significant pulmonary problems and may require maintenance of a controlled airway (via nasotracheal or endotracheal intubation) and assisted ventilation. Strict adherence to tracheobronchial hygiene is an important preventive measure in all patients, particularly those with limited pulmonary reserve. Encouraging deep breathing and coughing, use of humidified air to prevent inspissation of secretions and avoidance of oversedation are all indicated. Proper management of the patient on a mechanical ventilator requires frequent measurements of blood gases and appropriate correction of the ventilatory pattern when indicated (see Ventilatory Support, p. 85).

Since inadequate tissue oxygenation is a consistent feature of shock, attention to all components of the oxygen transport system is essential (see Oxygen Transport, p. 97). Efforts to maintain a normal or rightward positioned oxygen-hemoglobin dissociation curve may be particularly important in view of reported reductions in red blood cell organic phosphates in late septic shock.[22] The use of hyperbaric oxygen has also been suggested and would appear to be an ideal therapeutic approach. Limited experience with its use has been disappointing, however.[7, 21]

REFERENCES

1. Alican, F., Dalton, M. L., Jr., and Hardy, J. D.: Experimental endotoxin shock. Amer. J. Surg., *103*:702, 1962.
2. Altemeier, W. A., Todd, J. C., and Inge, W. W.: Gram-negative septicemia: A growing threat. Ann. Surg., *166*:530, 1967.
3. Ballet, S., and Kostis, J. B.: Recent Advances in the Therapy of Cardiac Arrhythmias. In: Cardiac Arrhythmias. A Symposium, Ed. J. Han. Springfield, Ill., Charles C Thomas, 1972, p. 260.
4. Baue, A. E.: The treatment of septic shock: A problem intensified by advancing science. Surgery, *65*:850, 1969.
5. Berk, J. L., Hagen, J. F., Beyer, W. H., Gerber, M. J., and Dochat, G. R.: The treatment of endotoxin shock by beta adrenergic blockade. Ann. Surg., *169*:74, 1969.
6. Berk, J. L., Hagen, J. F., and Dunn, J. M.: The role of beta adrenergic blockade in the treatment of septic shock. Surg., Gynec. Obstet., *130*:1025, 1970.
7. Blair, E., Ollodart, R., Esmond, W. G., Attar, S., and Cowley, R. A.: Effect of hyperbaric oxygenation (OHP) on bacteremic shock. Circulation (Suppl. I), *29*:135, 1964.
8. Carey, J. S., et al.: Cardiovascular function in shock: Responses to volume loading and isoproterenol infusion. Circulation, *35*:327, 1967.
9. Cook, W. A., Schwartz, D. L., and Bass, B. G.: Arfonad therapy: Hemodynamic responses and control. Ann. Thorac. Surg., *7*:322, 1969.

10. Duff, J. H., Malave, G., Pertz, D. I., Scott, H. M., and MacLean, L. D.: The hemo-dynamics of septic shock in man and in the dog. Surgery, 58:174, 1965.
11. Fitts, C. T.: Vasoactive drugs in treatment of shock. Postgrad. Med., 48:105, 1970.
12. Forrester, J. S., Diamond, G., McHugh, T. J., and Swan, H. J. C.: Filling pressures in the right and left sides of the heart in acute myocardial infarction. A reappraisal of central-venous-pressure monitoring. New Eng. J. Med., 285:190, 1971.
13. Freis, E. D., Schnaper, H. W., Johnson, R. L., and Schreiner, G. E.: Hemodynamic alterations in acute myocardial infarction. I. Cardiac output, mean arterial pressure, total peripheral resistance, "central" and total blood volumes, venous pressure and average circulation time. J. Clin. Invest., 31:131, 1952.
14. Grollman, A.: Cardiac Output of Man in Health and Disease. Springfield, Ill., Charles C Thomas, 1932.
15. Gunnar, R. M., and Loeb, H. S.: Use of drugs in cardiogenic shock due to acute myocardial infarction. Circulation, 45:1111, 1972.
16. Iampietro, P. F., Henshaw, L. B., and Brake, C. M.: Effect of an adrenergic blocking agent on vascular alterations associated with endotoxin shock. Amer. J. Physiol., 204:611, 1963.
17. Janoff, A., Weissman, G., Zweifach, B. W., and Thomas, L.: Pathogens of experi-mental shock. IV. Studies on lysosomes in normal and tolerant animals subjected to lethal trauma and endotoxemia. J. Exp. Med., 16:451, 1962.
18. Kouchoukos, N. T., Sheppard, L. C., and Kirklin, J. W.: Effect of alterations in arterial pressure on cardiac performance early after open intracardiac operations. J. Thorac. Cardiovasc. Surg., 64:563, 1972.
19. Kwaan, H. M., and Weil, M. H.: Differences in the mechanism of shock caused by bacterial infections. Surg., Gynec. Obstet., 128:37, 1969.
20. Lillehei, R. C., and MacLean, L. D.: Physiological approach to successful treatment of endotoxin shock in the experimental animal. Arch. Surg., 78:464, 1959.
21. MacLean, L. D., Mulligan, W. G., McLean, A. P. H., and Duff, J. H.: Patterns of septic shock in man — A detailed study of 56 patients. Ann. Surg., 166:543, 1967.
22. Miller, L. D., et al.: The affinity of hemoglobin for oxygen: Its control and in vivo significance. Surgery, 68:187, 1970.
23. Moore, D. C.: Complications of Regional Anesthesia. In: Clinical Anesthesia, Ed., J. J. Bonica. Philadelphia, F. A. Davis Company, 1969, p. 218.
24. Moss, G. S., Homer, L. D., Herman, C. M., and Proctor, H. J.: Right atrial and pulmonary artery pressure as indicators of left atrial pressure during fluid therapy following hemorrhagic shock in baboon. Ann. Surg., 170:801, 1969.
25. Motsay, G. J., Dietzman, R. H., Ersek, R. A., and Lillehei, R. C.: Hemodynamic alterations and results of treatment in patients with gram-negative septic shock. Surgery, 67:577, 1970.
26. Mueller, H., Ayres, S. M., Gregory, J. J., Giannelli, S., Jr., and Grace, W. J.: Hemo-dynamics, coronary blood flow, and myocardial metabolism in coronary shock: Re-sponse to I-norepinephrine and Isoproterenol. J. Clin. Invest., 49:1885, 1970.
27. Mullins, C. B., Sugg, W. L., Kennelly, B. M., Jones, D. C., and Mitchell, J. H.: Effect of arterial counterpulsation on left ventricular volume and pressure. Amer. J. Physiol., 220:694, 1971.
28. Ollodart, R. M., Hawthorne, I., and Attar, S.: Studies in experimental endotoxemia in man. Amer. J. Surg., 113:599, 1967.
29. Rahimtoola, S. H., et al.: Relationship of pulmonary artery to left ventricular di-astolic pressures in acute myocardial infarction. Circulation, 46:283, 1972.
30. Sanders, C. A., Buckley, M. J., Leinbach, R. C., Mundth, E. D., and Austen, W. G.: Mechanical circulatory assistance: Current status and experience with combining circulatory assistance, emergency, coronary angiography, and acute myocardial re-vascularization. Circulation, 45:1292, 1972.
31. Schumer, W., and Nyhus, L. M.: Corticosteroids in the Treatment of Shock. Ur-bana, Illinois, University of Illinois Press, Chicago, 1970.
32. Sharefkin, J. B., and MacArthur, J. D.: Pulmonary arterial pressure as a guide to the hemodynamic status of surgical patients. Arch. Surg., 105:699, 1972.
33. Shubin, H., and Weil, M. H.: Bacterial shock: A serious complication in urological practice. J.A.M.A., 185:850, 1963.

34. Spink, W. W.: The Ecology of Human Septic Shock. In: Septic Shock in Man, Ed. by Hershey, Del Guercio and McConn. Boston, Little, Brown and Co., 1971.
35. Spodick, D. H.: Acute cardiac tamponade. Pathologic physiology, diagnosis and management. Progr. Cardiovasc. Dis., 10:64, 1967.
36. Sugg, W. L., Rea, M. J., Webb, W. R., and Ecker, R. R.: Cardiac assistance (counter-pulsation) in ten patients. Clinical and hemodynamic observations. Ann. Thorac. Surg., 9:1, 1970.
37. Swan, H. J. C., et al.: Catheterization of the heart in man with use of a flow-directed balloon-tipped catheter. New Eng. J. Med., 283:447, 1970.
38. Waldhausen, J. A., Kilman, J. W., and Abel, F. L.: Effects of catecholamines on the heart. Myocardial contractility, cardiac efficiency, and total peripheral resistance. Arch. Surg., 91:86, 1965.
39. Weil, M. H., Shubin, H., and Rosoff, L.: Fluid repletion in circulatory shock: Central venous pressure and other practical guides. J.A.M.A., 192:668, 1965.
40. Wilson, J. N., Grow, J. B., Demong, C. V., Prevedel, A. E., and Owens, J. C.: Central venous pressure in optimal blood volume maintenance. Arch. Surg., 85:563, 1962.
41. Wilson, R. F., and Fisher, R. R.: The hemodynamic effects of massive steroids in clinical shock. Surg., Gynec. Obstet., 127:769, 1968.
42. Wilson, R. F., Sukhnanden, R., and Thal, A. P.: Combined use of norepinephrine and dibenzyline in clinical shock. Surg. Forum, 15:30, 1964.

Index

Note: Page numbers in *italics* indicate illustrations; (t) refers to tables.

Adrenergic mechanisms, *136*
Alkalosis, resuscitation and, in post-
traumatic pulmonary insufficiency, 62
Antibiotics, in hypovolemic shock, 128
in pulmonary insufficiency, 92
in septic shock, 156
Aspiration of gastric contents, in
pulmonary insufficiency, 70

Blood flow, low rate of, 10
Blood pressure, changes in shock, 5(t),
6, 7, *29*, *31*
Blood substitutes, 125
Blood transfusions, 104
and DPG levels, 105(t), *106*
in hemorrhagic shock, 108
therapeutic implications of, 109, *121*
Blood urea nitrogen (BUN) values, 44, *44*,
50
after renal ischemia, 57
in high-output renal failure, 51, *52*

Cardiac output, after trauma, *46*
Cardiogenic shock, 145–149
catecholamines in, 147
digitalis in, 147
ganglionic blockade in, 148
hemodynamic measurements in, 145
mechanical assistance for, 149
Catecholamines, in cardiogenic shock, 147
Cerebral injury, as cause of pulmonary
insufficiency, 76
Circulation, in post-traumatic pulmonary
insufficiency, 62
Classification of shock, 4
Clinical manifestations of shock, 1–12
Colloid administration, as cause of
pulmonary insufficiency, 73
Compliance, changes in, in pulmonary
insufficiency, 84

Constant positive-pressure breathing
(CPPB), 87
Contractility, myocardial, abnormalities
in, 147

Digitalis, in cardiogenic shock, 147
in hypovolemic shock, 129
in septic shock, 159
2,3-Diphosphoglycerate (DPG), and
blood transfusions, 104, 105(t), *106*,
109
and oxygen-hemoglobin dissociation
curve, 102, *103*
Diuretics, in pulmonary insufficiency, 91
Drug therapy, in pulmonary insufficiency,
90. See also specific types of drugs, as
Digitalis, Steroids etc.

Electrolytes, extracellular and
intracellular, 27, 30(t), 31(t), *32*, *34*, *35*,
36, *37*, *38*
Embolization, fat, 71. See also
Microembolization.
Epinephrine, levels in shock, 9. See also
Catecholamines.
Extracellular fluid, measurement of, 17,
18
replacement in hemorrhagic shock, 120
response of, 15–41

Fat embolization, 71
Fluid electrolytes, overload, and
pulmonary function, 72
Fluid management, in pulmonary
insufficiency, 89
Fluid overload, 72
Fluid replacement, in hemorrhagic shock,
120
in septic shock, 157

163

Ganglionic blockade, in cardiogenic shock, 148
Glomerular filtration rate (GFR), 43, *45*, 47, 49

Heart, abnormal ventricular rates in, 148
Hematocrit, in hemorrhagic shock, 124, *125*
Hemodilution, 8
Hemodynamic measurements, 138–141
  in cardiogenic shock, 145
Hemoglobin concentration, in pulmonary insufficiency, 86
Hemorrhagic shock, 16. See also *Hypovolemic shock.*
  action potentials in, *32, 33*
  blood replacement in, 120
  blood transfusions in, 108
  blood urea nitrogen levels in, *55*
  cellular studies in, 18
    interpretation of, 33
  extracellular fluid replacement in, 120
  fluid electrolyte changes in, 31(t), *32, 34, 35, 36, 37, 38*
  hematocrit in, 124, *125*
  in ischemic pulmonary injury, 65
  interstitial fluid response in, *19*, 21
  intrapulmonary shunting after, *66*
  lactate levels in, 121, *122, 123*
  survival studies in, *17*
  urine volume in, *55*
Heparin, in pulmonary insufficiency, 91
Hypercarbia with asystole, in post-traumatic pulmonary insufficiency, 63
Hypocarbia, 87
Hypothermia, in hypovolemic shock, 130
    technique of, 131
  renal, in hypovolemic shock, 130, *132, 133, 134, 135*
Hypoventilation, 77
Hypovolemic shock, 119–144. See also *Hemorrhagic shock.*
  antibiotics in, 128
  digitalis in, 129
  experimental studies in, 15
  hypothermia in, 130
    technique of, 131
  intra-arterial infusions for, 129
  positioning of patient in, 126
  pulmonary support in, 127
  steroids in, 129
  treatment of pain in, 128
  vasodilators in, 137
  vasopressors in, 135
Hypoxemia, causes of, 78(t)
Hypoxia, 77
  terminal, in post-traumatic pulmonary insufficiency, 63

Intermittent positive-pressure breathing (IPPB), 85
Interstitial fluid response, in hemorrhagic shock, *19*, 21
Ion transport, 19
Ischemia, renal, effect of hypothermia on, 56

Kidney, responses to shock, 42–60. See also *Renal.*

Lactate levels, in hemorrhagic shock, 121, *122, 123*
Ling-Gerard ultramicroelectrode, 19, *20*
Lung volumes and capacities, *78*

Measurements, hemodynamic, 138–141
  in cardiogenic shock, 145
Membrane potential. See under *Muscle, skeletal.*
Metabolic changes, 10, 48
Microatelectasis, in post-traumatic pulmonary insufficiency, 76
Microembolization, 71
Muscle, skeletal, membrane potential in, 26, *29*, 30(t), *32, 35*
Myocardial contractility, abnormalities in, 147

Neurogenic shock, 149–150

Oxygen pressure, arterial, 83
Oxygen toxicity, in post-traumatic pulmonary insufficiency, 75
Oxygen transport, alterations in, 97–115
    following transfusion, 104–109
Oxygen transport system, 97–99
Oxygenation, evaluation of, in post-traumatic pulmonary insufficiency, 82
Oxygen-hemoglobin dissociation curve, 99, *100, 108, 113*
  factors influencing, 101, 102(t)

Pain, treatment of, in hypovolemic shock, 128
Para-aminohippurate (PAH) clearances, 43
Pathophysiologic responses, 13–115

Patient monitoring, in post-traumatic pulmonary insufficiency, 82
Pco$_2$, control of, 87
pH, of blood, 10
Pituitary-adrenal changes, 9
Positioning of patient, in hypovolemic shock, 126
Post-traumatic pulmonary insufficiency, 61
  diagnosis of, 64(t)
  etiology of, 64
  hemorrhagic shock in, 65
  phases of, 62
Potassium. See also *Electrolytes.*
Potassium levels, 10, 11
"Primary shock." See *Neurogenic shock.*
Primate studies, 25, 33
Pulmonary capillary permeability, measurement of, 74, *74*, 75(t)
Pulmonary care, in pulmonary insufficiency, 90
Pulmonary injury, as cause of pulmonary insufficiency, 76
Pulmonary insufficiency, etiology of, 64–77
  post-traumatic, clinical presentation of, 62–64
    aspiration of gastric contents in, 70
    diagnosis of, 64(t)
    etiology of, 64–77
    mechanism of, 77–80
    patient study protocol for, 67(t)
    phases of, 62
    progressive, 63
    sepsis in, 70
      incidence of, 68(t)
    treatment of, 80–92
Pulmonary responses, 61–96
Pulmonary support, in hypovolemic shock, 127
  in post-traumatic pulmonary insufficiency, 85
  complications, 88
Pulmonary therapy, in septic shock, 160
Pulse rate, changes in shock, 5(t), 7

Renal damage, subclinical, following injury and shock, 42
Renal failure, high output, 50
  blood urea nitrogen values in, 51, *52*
  carbon dioxide-combining power in, *54*
  serum potassium levels in, *53*
  serum sodium levels in, *54*
  urine volume in, *52*
  nonoliguric. See *Renal failure, high-output.*
Renal function, after trauma, 43(t), *44*, *45*
Renal hypothermia, in hypovolemic shock, 130, *132*, *133*, *134*, *135*

Renal ischemia, blood urea values following, 57
  effect of hypothermia on, 56
Renal responses, 42–60
Respiration, difficult, in post-traumatic pulmonary insufficiency, 62
Resuscitation and alkalosis, in post-traumatic pulmonary insufficiency, 62

Sepsis, gram-negative, and shock, 152
  associated conditions and, 152
  bacteriology of, 153
  clinical manifestations of, 153
  source of, 152
  treatment of, 156
  gram-positive, and shock, 151
  in post-traumatic pulmonary insufficiency, 70
Septic shock, 151–160. See also *Sepsis.*
Shock, biochemical changes in, 9
  cardiogenic, 145–149. See also *Cardiogenic shock.*
  classification of, 4
  clinical manifestations of, 1–12
  definition of, 3
  grading of, 5(t)
  hemorrhagic, 16. See also *Hemorrhagic shock.*
  hypovolemic, 119–144. See also *Hypovolemic shock.*
  neurogenic, 149–150
  organ failure in, 11
  pathophysiologic responses to, 13–115
  physiologic changes in, 7
  septic, 151–160. See also *Sepsis.*
"Shock lung," classic, 66, 68(t), 69(t)
Shunting, intrapulmonary, after hemorrhagic shock, *66*
  pulmonary, causes of, *79*
Skin changes, in shock, 5(t)
Small animal studies, 19
Sodium. See *Electrolytes.*
Steroids, in hypovolemic shock, 129
  in pulmonary insufficiency, 91
  in septic shock, 156

Thirst, in shock, 5(t), 6
Trauma, cardiac output after, *46*
  renal function after, 43(t), *44*, *45*

Urine/plasma urea ratio, *45*, 49
Urine volume, in high-output renal failure, *52*

Vasoconstriction, 8
Vasodilators, in hypovolemic shock, 137
  in septic shock, 159
Vasopressors, in hypovolemic shock, 135
  in septic shock, 158
Ventilation, evaluation of, in post-
  traumatic pulmonary insufficiency, 84

Ventilation-perfusion ratio, 79
Ventilatory reserve, 84
Ventilatory support, in post-traumatic
  pulmonary insufficiency, 85
  complications, 88